Conundrums of Care

New Writing in Critical Development Studies series, edited by Wendy Harcourt

New Writing in Critical Development Studies brings together new critical and alternative development research by established and early career researchers from around the world. Foregrounding postdevelopment, decoloniality, political ecology, feminism, antiracism, pluriversality, and related concepts and approaches, the series provides a vehicle for emerging trends in critical development scholarship. The series is distinctive for its dedication to publishing new writers, particularly those based in the Global South, alongside more canonical voices. It is also uniquely open to alternative forms of knowledge production, including photographs, drawings, figures, and other artwork. Books are academically rigorous, but also concise and readable, making them ideal for researchers from diverse disciplinary backgrounds, as well as for students, practitioners, activists, and policymakers.

Conundrums of Care

Feminist Entanglements in Critical Development Studies

Wendy Harcourt

BLOOMSBURY ACADEMIC
LONDON • NEW YORK • OXFORD • NEW DELHI • SYDNEY

BLOOMSBURY ACADEMIC
Bloomsbury Publishing Plc, 50 Bedford Square, London, WC1B 3DP, UK
Bloomsbury Publishing Inc, 1359 Broadway, New York, NY 10018, USA
Bloomsbury Publishing Ireland, 29 Earlsfort Terrace, Dublin 2, D02 AY28, Ireland

BLOOMSBURY, BLOOMSBURY ACADEMIC and the Diana logo are trademarks of Bloomsbury Publishing Plc

First published in Great Britain 2025

Copyright © Wendy Harcourt, 2025

Wendy Harcourt has asserted her right under the Copyright, Designs and Patents Act, 1988, to be identified as Author of this work.

For legal purposes the Acknowledgements on p. xii constitute an extension of this copyright page.

Cover image: Embrace by Emma Claire Sardoni

All rights reserved. No part of this publication may be: i) reproduced or transmitted in any form, electronic or mechanical, including photocopying, recording or by means of any information storage or retrieval system without prior permission in writing from the publishers; or ii) used or reproduced in any way for the training, development or operation of artificial intelligence (AI) technologies, including generative AI technologies. The rights holders expressly reserve this publication from the text and data mining exception as per Article 4(3) of the Digital Single Market Directive (EU) 2019/790.

Bloomsbury Publishing Plc does not have any control over, or responsibility for, any third-party websites referred to or in this book. All internet addresses given in this book were correct at the time of going to press. The author and publisher regret any inconvenience caused if addresses have changed or sites have ceased to exist, but can accept no responsibility for any such changes.

A catalogue record for this book is available from the British Library.

Library of Congress Cataloging-in-Publication Data available

ISBN:	HB:	978-1-3504-5960-1
	PB:	978-1-3504-5959-5
	ePDF:	978-1-3504-5962-5
	eBook:	978-1-3504-5961-8

Typeset by RefineCatch Limited, Bungay, Suffolk
Printed and bound in Great Britain

For product safety related questions contact productsafety@bloomsbury.com.

To find out more about our authors and books visit www.bloomsbury.com and sign up for our newsletters.

For Pancho, a sweet and caring more-than-human companion

Contents

Preface		ix
Acknowledgements		xii
1	Caring Conversations: An Introduction	1
	What we explore in this chapter	1
	Section One: *Lake stories*	2
	Section Two: *Vignettes*	9
	Section Three: *Meaning making*	23
	Conundrums of caring conversations	29
2	Care Work: Valuing Social Reproduction	31
	What we explore in this chapter	31
	Section One: *Pandemic crisis stories*	32
	Section Two: *Valuing care work*	36
	Section Three: *Feminist recovery plans and manifestos*	49
	Conundrums of care work	53
3	Earthcare: Ecofeminist and Indigenous Approaches to Our Life-worlds	55
	What we explore in this chapter	55
	Section One: *Stories of Earthcare*	55
	Section Two: *Earthothers*	61
	Section Three: *Intercultural weavings*	69
	Conundrums of Earthcare	76
4	Caring about Having Babies: Reproductive Rights and Population Ethics	79
	What we explore in this chapter	79
	Section One: *Birth stories*	80
	Section Two: *The choice to parent*	83

	Section Three: *Kinning*	89
	Conundrums of having babies	96
5	Interspecies Care: Learning with the More-than-Human	97
	What we explore in this chapter	97
	Section One: *Companion stories*	97
	Section Two: *Interspecies entanglements*	100
	Section Three: *Embodied toxicity*	109
	Conundrums of interspecies care	117
6	Caring Communities: Building Reciprocity through Degrowth, Community Economies and Radical Care	119
	What we explore in this chapter	119
	Section One: *Caring encounters*	120
	Section Two: *Community economies and commoning*	124
	Section Three: *Radical care*	134
	Conundrums of radical care	143
7	Connecting with Care: Pedagogies for Transformation	147
	What we explore in this chapter	147
	Section One: *Teaching with care*	147
	Section Two: *Careful disruptions*	151
	Section Three: *Repositioning care*	159
	Conundrums of connecting with care	164
Epilogue		167
Notes		171
References		183
Index		207

Preface

While I have been thinking about what it means to care as a feminist activist, mother, teacher, advocate and researcher for years, I didn't find the courage to start writing this book for a long time. There was always the troubling voice in my head saying, 'who are you to be writing about care?' I suffered from the usual imposter syndrome of academe. I was acutely aware that there were many other points of view that deserved to be heard rather than mine. Even once I got the contract to write the book, I was dithering around until I attended an Avron writing retreat in Lumb Bank, West Yorkshire.

This was a life writing retreat held in an eighteenth-century house once owned by Ted Hughes (and near where Sylvia Plath is buried). It promised to be a dream week. My room, with its simple desk set against a large window, looked down a velvety green valley. Even the September rain couldn't dim the prettiness of the place. We ate delicious meals concocted from food grown in the garden. Cakes were made and served every afternoon. After a morning of writing exercises, we would be given ample time to ply away on our projects or take walks in the valley ready to report progress in the evenings, after more delectable food. I was relieved I was not the oldest attending, nor the only person who had made a living as an editor or worked in international development. But notably, I was the only academic. This proved to be the key to what was making me feel the odd one out. Whereas everyone else was happily sharing their writings, chatting about their book projects and exchanging their life stories as we walked briskly around the hills in the mud and rain, I was nervously wondering not only about my competence, but also about my political position to write anything at all.

One evening we were gathered around the fire in the front room. People had bought some bottles of red from the local pub and the plan was to read out what we had written that day while we sipped wine. I was not at all sure I was going to participate. I had found it hard to engage in the morning's writing exercise. I had been called on to speak by one of the tutors as he said I rarely volunteered. I had felt shamed, but when I read out what I had written, his only comment was that I had an extensive vocabulary. I found myself feeling judged and was wondering if this retreat had been a good idea after all, despite the views and the food. I was not at all keen to share what I had written that afternoon. In fact, I was just about to slip out of the room when one of the men called over to me that people were curious what I had been writing when they had gone down to the pub. The others looked up expectantly. Their kind faces and the cheeriness of the room, with the fire and colourful bookshelves, made me pause and I sat down.

Eventually, after a glass of wine, I found myself sharing how hard it was to write as a white older Australian activist turned academic living in Europe about topics I felt passionate about. Who was I to write about care when I had so much privilege and luck and really it was other peoples' stories that were interesting, not mine? They looked surprised and then thoughtful. 'But we all have our own stories to tell, right?' said one of the women a little older than me (who it transpired had been in a travelling circus at some point in her life). 'And it sounds like your life with all that international travel and meetings is interesting enough.' But was I writing about my life I wondered?

We then had a long discussion about how academic writing pretended knowledge was not formed by the author's life experiences in its claim to be objective. They convinced me that story writing was also about producing knowledge. Why not reveal more about how I had gained the knowledge I wanted to share and why it was inspiring for me? Instead of culling ideas into dry facts, why not present them as stories? Why not be transparent about why I found the people or place or encounter interesting? It was then up to the reader to decide if what I wrote was interesting for them. They also told me that academic writing was not aspirational, too often full of jargon. They suggested I find ways to write that build on experience and are clear and easy to follow.

At the end of the retreat, I found the courage to share something I had written that afternoon while staring out the window down the valley. It was a story about one of my visits to Jaipur, India to give lectures on gender and development and the conundrum of care I felt when I was taken by one of my hosts to visit a local fabric shop. While being shown the cottons and silks, I saw through the doorway a dozen young women wearing brightly coloured saris seated in rows working away at old Singer sewing machines. When I went to speak to them to acknowledge their work and learn more about their lives, the foreman seated at the spotless front desk waved me over to explain they only spoke the local *Dhundari*. I exchanged silent smiles with the women and turned away. I felt troubled as I dutifully bought the patterned wood block cotton shirts and blouses to take home as gifts. In the story I tried to explain the yawning gap between the lives of those women and my own, but how still I cared about the entanglement of our lives, even if they touched just for a moment. I wanted to share what I felt about the meanings of care, privilege, work and difference of culture, class, race, ethnicity, age. While the book has gone on to explore other entanglements than the specific conundrum I felt in Jaipur, sharing the story encouraged by the care of my fellow writers at the retreat served as its beginning. I hope that you enjoy the stories, and that you *do* find them interesting.

Acknowledgements

Thank you to my feminist friends, allies and students who have inspired me over the years. Special thanks to Di, Linda, Agustina, Alex, Ayesha, Franck, Emma Claire and Roy, who read earlier versions of various chapters and who listened patiently to my ideas and encouraged me to keep going.

Thank you also to my colleagues of the WEGO-ITN network, the International Institute of Social Studies, the Erasmus University Rotterdam library and Bloomsbury Academic who provided the wherewithal for me to write and publish the book.

1

Caring Conversations: An Introduction

The act of sharing stories is the theory and the methodology.
Katherine McKittrick 2021: 73.

What we explore in this chapter

This first chapter starts with a story spun from my life-sustaining connections with *il Lago di Bolsena* (Bolsena Lake) in central Italy. By the shores of the lake, I have holidayed with family and friends, held writing retreats and workshops and spent many hours walking, swimming and dreaming. After the story I present a series of 'Vignettes'. They are snapshots of how my understandings of care are guided by my life-experiences and feminist activism. A third section on 'Meaning Making' presents my feminist influences and the methodological approach to the book and how I understand care broadly speaking as the life-making and life-sustaining activities that maintain humans and more-than-humans in our life-worlds. My interest is in care for processes – social, political, ecological, corporeal – in the more expansive sense of the Latin word for care, *curatus*, where the gendered nature of care work is historically contextualised (rather than essentialised) as female. As with all chapters I conclude with a reflection on the conundrums I have raised in the chapter, in this case anticipating some of the book's recurring conundrums of care.

Section One: *Lake stories*

The first time I saw the deep blue lake glinting through the trees it felt like magic. Now eighteen years later that first view, as the car winds down the hill on the road from Rome to Bolsena, still lifts my heart and draws me in. I care deeply about the blue volcanic lake, 100 or so kilometres north of Rome. As I move in and out of the community nestled around it, I feel the depth of its Etruscan past and the promise of its evolving future entangled with mine. Something in the place has captured me. In the years since I first glimpsed the lake, I have joined and hosted various workshops and retreats; held my fiftieth birthday party one cold but glorious spring weekend; bought a tiny little house perched on top of the castle walls with its sweeping panoramic view; swum in folds of silken lake waters during hot August mornings; and invited many people to come to its shores to learn, dream and celebrate creating community with me.

Though it still feels magical, caring for *Lago di Bolsena* is not straightforward. The community is traditionally conservative, with centuries of church and local aristocratic families dominating its economy and politics. Individuals from outside come and go. The traditional cultures of farming and small tourist-based businesses have little time for outsiders. There is however something of a counterculture, celebrating the local food, music and artisanal crafts. For over a decade, I belonged to a small community organisation based in the town's seventeenth-century Franciscan *Convento* (monastery). We would host workshops and cultural festivals. Sadly, our little network unravelled during Covid-19 in 2020 and the community association fell apart. The local music and art festivals which were hosted by the town in the summers are notably fewer as post-Covid-19 recession bites. The small family restaurants struggle to keep going. The lake is becoming more polluted as climate change means the winter winds are no longer fierce or durable enough to clean the lake. Fracking in a nearby town is threatening to break open the lake boundaries. The increasingly hot summers mean fewer fish and more algae. There is little state money coming into Bolsena to keep the pumps around the lake working, and sewerage seeps in from hotels and camp sites. Locals rarely swim in the lake now.

Stories of care interweave throughout my times in Bolsena. To begin, I share a story from the early days of my relations with Bolsena's life-worlds as a first kernel of the conundrums of care I explore in this book.

During the long Italian summers I spent in Bolsena, I would annually organise workshops at the *Convento*. The Franciscan order, which owns the *Convento*, gave usufructuary rights (with no rent) to the association, with the proviso that pilgrims walking the *Francigena* path (from Canterbury to Rome) would be hosted at the *Convento*. Even with the order's generosity, volunteers are needed to keep the place running. Old walls crumble, plumbing erodes, rooms and kitchens require new furnishings. So, like many small community organisations, chasing money was the order of the day.

In the late 2000s I was invited to facilitate a UN panel on gender and food security in the gleaming glass headquarters of the International Fund for Agricultural Development (IFAD) on the outskirts of Rome. I took up the invitation largely to see if there was any possibility of financial support for the community organisation. I anticipated a series of talks delivered by gender experts about their projects working with struggling women farmers in villages in Asia and Africa. At the meeting I had no luck with funding, but I did encounter a fellow feminist traveller – Parto, an Iranian feminist academic working at the Humboldt University in Berlin. She stood out with her characteristically (as I came to find out) bright dresses and scarves in vivid primary colours. Her eyes flashed with passion about her work. Through photos and Iranian women's art – in stark contrast to the dull PowerPoints of the other speakers – she explained enthusiastically about the concept of 'meal cultures'. The concept emerged from her research with economically marginal women struggling to find food security in villages in Iran, Sudan and Kenya. She used the term meal culture rather than food security to recognise the importance of the time and care taken by women not only to produce edible food, but also to create family and community lives around meals. She argued that food security, in its deeper sense, should not just be about access to food stuffs, it should also be about the time and labour required to prepare, serve and bring people together at mealtimes. Meals are a microcosm of complex social, cultural and gender relations. People do not eat meat, cereal or vegetables raw. It is mostly women (of a certain age, class and status in the community) who do the material, social and cultural work of meal preparation. In every culture there are rules around what kind of food can be served when, who does the cooking, who serves, how much each person is expected to eat according to gender, age and the occasion. There is an order (implicit or explicit) of where people sit, and the timing of who eats when, whether it is all together or first older men or young children. The focus of experts on the economics of agricultural provisioning of food ignores the everyday care work of women to prepare meals and the cultural and social care taken around meals. Parto argued that understanding the care work that went into meals is necessary to secure the future of sustainable food systems and food business.

After her talk, I introduced myself. I was eager to find out more about her concept of meal cultures. We missed several of the other panels as we chatted in the corner drinking tiny Italian espresso coffees, excitedly discussing how to explore meal cultures in Europe. I immediately suggested we could host a workshop at the *Convento* in Bolsena. Parto was keen to explore meal cultures among Berlin's food networks. When we left the meeting, we embraced and said how much we both looked forward to future collaboration.

A year later we had applied and received funding from the EU *Grundtvig* programme (part of the *European* Commission's Lifelong Learning Programme from 2007–2013) allowing us to hold two workshops, one in Bolsena and one in Berlin. At the Bolsena workshop we brought together fifteen women and a couple of men from around West and East Europe to share their meal cultures. During our week together, we visited the family farms around Bolsena and invited older women who lived in a nearby village to demonstrate how to make *pici*, a traditional eggless pasta from *Tuscia*, the area around the lake. We cooked meals and ate together under the vines outside the *Convento*'s large kitchen watching the sunset over the lake. We prepared and enjoyed tasting cheese pies from Turkey, potato dishes from the Ukraine, beet stews from Bulgaria and apple strudels from Germany. We visited Orvieto to learn about the slow food movement and the impending sense of encroachment of EU regulations on traditional foods threatening small family farms. We tasted wines made by three sisters who had inherited their grandfather's farm. We ate fish from the lake, enjoyed delicious ice-cream made in local factories nearby and sampled the different sheep's cheese made by families from Sardinia who had settled in the *Tuscia* area. It was a bucolic moment that honoured the different meal cultures by eating together and listening to the different stories of change. The lake gleamed in the background. A group of us went swimming each morning when the lake was like a vast blue mirror. We shared simple stories based on recipes that were proffered as part of meal cultures that were embedded in places around Europe. The idea of meal cultures was only loosely linked to the bigger political issues around food security. Our embodied and gendered lives were connected via the practice of preparing and eating meals together. The purpose was to come together for a week and to learn from our experiences, enjoy communal meal preparations and experience the lake and *Tuscia* region and learn about some of the different meal cultures found in Europe.

In contrast, our workshop in Berlin with around twenty-five people was more intentionally political and academic by design. We stayed in Humboldt University digs in East Berlin, and traversed the city by train and tram to experience a vast assortment of meal cultures. We visited a Church organisation that collected food waste and ate the left-over food binned by supermarkets, cooking soup together with homeless people who came every night to eat. We met a glamorous local TV chef and sampled her desserts off-camera. We visited environmental groups who were campaigning against fast food and plastic food packaging. We met with migrant groups from Turkey who served us flat bread and soft white cheese for lunch, and others from former German African colonies, who served us hot curries, plantains and chai. At the university we met lecturers who explained about global food politics. One night we cooked an elaborate Iranian meal supervised by an elegant friend of Parto's who taught cooking professionally. We gathered in her huge house to learn about three ways to cook rice and to prepare vegetables which we had bought earlier in an open-air market. Her kitchen gleamed with expansive ovens, deep sinks, marble tops and an impressive array of pans, pots and other cooking implements. The rich variety of meal cultures in Berlin was a far cry from the tours around rural Bolsena and our meals prepared together in the convent kitchen with its odd assortment of plates, battered metal pots and mismatched plates.

These complex connections of care which spooled from that first meeting with Parto provide a hint at the conundrums of care we will be exploring in the book. As entrepreneurial intellectuals and as passionate and caring feminists, Parto and I made good use of two European-funded events to explore meal cultures involving our networks. Our story flowed from the lake into a UN building and out into the lives of people in networks across Europe. This process is how, from my experience, feminism as a caring process works in privileged settings where there is access to funds, creating spaces through trust, forging connections beyond institutionalised spaces, finding ways to share ideas and connecting in non-institutionalised ways. (As well as learning how to write convincing funding proposals for feminist networking and campaigns.) At the heart of these two stories is the visceral and embodied experience of preparing meals, learning about meal cultures, and a desire to build knowledge and community from (mostly female) gendered everyday experiences. We connected in both a rural and urban setting to young and old feminists, farmers, wine makers, cheese makers, migrant communities, older rural women, environmentalists, TV cooks, religious institutions and academics. The lake and the *Tuscia* area provided a rural setting where traditions and histories could be explored slowly and intentionally, where natural beauty, enjoyment of food and community mattered. In Berlin we had the urban experience of meal cultures created by a multi-cultural environment that thrived on an intoxicating mix of different peoples, cultures and types of food.

These stories reveal how the sharing of knowledge and experience of meals as a caring practice is as diverse as it is complex. There are overlaying histories and traditions in the different places and cultures. There is care shown in preparing and sharing the meals that reflects differential access to resources and different responsibilities around food processes, including food waste. The care taken in preparing meals is embedded in historical, cultural and social knowledge practices. The older women who taught us how to prepare *pici* in the convent kitchen come from peasant traditions passed on down the generations. Their knowledge and skill is gleaned from unpaid labour in the kitchens. *Pici* evolves from peasant needs to make affordable food from flour and water without eggs. The time taken, and the care put into making the pasta, means it was traditionally reserved for special occasions, as the time was taken away from other tasks. The value is in the time and care taken for others, rather than the actual economic cost of the flour. Reflecting this, the older women refused to be paid money for their demonstrations in the convent kitchen. They said they were pleased that foreigners wanted to know how to make *pici* and enjoyed eating our attempts sitting outside in the sun with us at the end of the afternoon. In contrast, the TV cook in Berlin producing home-made desserts on television displays her care for making desserts as a skill. Her performance is valued economically and socially. We paid for her time and the desserts we ate.

Our exploration of meal cultures shows how the practice of care is also political. The environmental campaigners in Berlin protesting at food waste measure and report on the waste created by plastic packaging as well as food being binned by supermarkets. Through their reports to political parties and municipalities they advocate for change at the local level. They combine this advocacy with local action collecting and transporting food waste from supermarkets to the homeless shelters, where volunteers sort food to be used for soups and stews and serve it to homeless people who gather every evening. These political actions show care for local communities and the environment.

Care is noticeably a gendered practice. While we met with some young men, the cooks in both Bolsena and Berlin were women, and the volunteers in the Church shelter were mostly older women. Most of our group were also women. It seemed that care taken in providing meals was the responsibility of women. Our project was paying attention to and honouring that care work. At the same time, as feminist academics at Humboldt University noted, care work could be oppressive. There were everyday humdrum practices that went into preparing meals, shopping, setting tables, washing dishes, cleaning, and repeat. The responsibility to do the cooking, including keeping the cultural heritage of elaborate food preparation, mostly falls on (unpaid labour) of women. It took time away from other more enjoyable or productive activities. We debated if we could revalue care. The care taken making and serving meals, providing nutrition and enjoyment for families and communities is trivialised as women's work. Care in these attitudes is gendered in a negative way as something female partners, sisters, daughters, mothers, grandmothers or female volunteers do in homes, charities and religious organisations – all institutions traditionally oppressive for women, according to their access to resources, knowledge, class, ethnic group, race and status. Yet these acts of care are vital, and need to be noticed and valued as we go through the conundrums of care.

And what, you may well ask, does my love of a lake have to do with all of this? Why am I sharing a story about a Grundtvig project in Bolsena and Berlin? Ah, this is where the personal is political. In the next section I share with you some vignettes which help position how my understanding of care has been shaped personally and politically, before discussing in the final section the meaning-making of care that undergirds the various chapters in the book.

Section Two: *Vignettes*

These following vignettes position my reflections on care in my personal and political embodied life. They help to explain how the book is informed by my lived feminist practice as well as my engagement with feminist theory. They reveal how the book emerges from the interweaving of my activism, advocacy, networking and teaching, which are reflected in the choices of where I lived and worked, with whom I partner and kin as an educated able-bodied white cis-woman who has enjoyed several decades of adulthood.

Vignette One: Balancing paid and unpaid care work

Balancing paid work and care work in the home for me involved juggling not only family and childcare but also continuous travel and keeping home in two countries. My two daughters were born in the late 1990s. I have an older male partner, who was continually being congratulated by his fellow academics for 'allowing' me to work. Apart from raising my feminist hackles, this observation was a total misnomer as living in cosmopolitan Rome, with no wider family support, we both needed to have incomes. As a woman of my time, I was determined to always earn, which meant working while having children. I also loved children and was equally determined to enjoy being a parent. In our family I took on the job of doing and organising the care work. The paid job I could find in Rome as an educated English-speaking foreigner was in the development aid sector. For over twenty years I edited a journal and ran advocacy and research programmes for an International NGO on various aspects of development – such as gender, health and environment. This required almost monthly travel. While my two daughters were under three years old (in Italy children go to elementary school when they turn three), we hired a young Filipina woman to look after them. She stayed to care for the family from when my younger daughter was one year old until both the children went to university. I met her via my gender and development networks. Most of my salary went into her wages. We ensured she had a legal contract including holidays and pension payments and maternity leave (she now has two sons). Ironically, though I had a job which I chose and could use my education, I was not given the choice to have such a contract – as was common in Italy in those days – NGOs were seen as closer to charities than as professional entities. Though I did not have a legally correct contract, I was thankful to be paid enough to cover childcare and I could organise the daily and often long-distance management of my family's care needs with someone who stayed with us for many years.

There are many conundrums here which need unpacking. There is the question of why I was willing to work without a legally correct contract? It was partly because I suffered from first world guilt about being paid to do work with people living in the Global South who were paid far less. I felt it unfair to demand a legal contract which would cost my organisation more. Second, why did I hire someone else from the Philippines to look after my daughters? The short answer was that I wanted someone who spoke English and who I met via my advocacy work. The other reality was that I was ineligible for state-run nurseries, and I could not afford (nor did I entirely trust) private nurseries. I juggled care work needs by working from home as much as possible and travelling with my daughters while I was breast-feeding. I was concerned about the sharing of family care in an economically and socially unequal situation, however much I tried to be fair, systemically as a white educated woman I definitely had the edge. How did I deal with this emotionally? Juggling paid work and care work took an emotional toll. I felt huge unease at not having a family or close-knit community to call on to help and at having to pay others for care work. At times I felt by doing paid work, especially travelling, I was letting down my daughters, who were an important and integral part of my life. When I took up academic work which did give me a legal contract, it meant I had to move to The Netherlands, away from family for long stretches of time. But at least I could discuss my reasons with my daughters, who were by then in their teens and twenties.

In Chapter 2 I go deeper into these conundrums around care work, reflecting on global care chains and what the Covid-19 pandemic crisis has taught us about the cost of undervaluing care work. Among others, I am inspired by Joan Tronto's work on moral ethics of care, the feminist economist Nancy Folbre on paid and unpaid work and philosopher Elke Krasny's book on care during Covid-19.

Vignette Two: Care for Earthothers

When I was eight years old, I painted a picture of a possum and her joeys with the caption: 'Will your grandchildren see them?' for a poster competition. It won and I was thrilled to see the picture in our local Sunday paper – but I was puzzled by the comment under the picture that my sentiment was particularly endearing because, after all, possums are pests. In Australia in those days, you could hire pest exterminators to deal with the possums running riot in your roof. Now under the 1975 Wildlife Act and subsequent acts, possums are legally protected, and you are fined if you harm them in any way. You are advised to close the roof cavity instead of killing possums. There are possum handlers rather than exterminators who are licensed to capture and release possums.

There are several stories of possums from my Australian childhood. There was the possum that fell through the roof of my uncle's dilapidated house into his tomato soup. I was not there but I have a vivid picture in my mind of the splash, the stained red walls and scramble that ensued as my uncle chased the intruder out of the kitchen. My father was particularly against possums as they would steal the eggs from the quails running around in his aviaries. Now I am slightly aghast at how we felt it was ok to have caged budgerigars and canaries inside our house and outside in the aviaries, galas, lorikeets and rosellas along with the quails (I explore this further in the story opening Chapter 5). We had several visits by the pest exterminators to get rid of possums. I remember visiting a farm up North and being proudly shown the possum skins by a teenage boy who had been allowed to shoot them as they were eating the fruit from the trees in the family's garden.

These childhood memories bring up several conundrums of care. How can humans live with more-than-human life, or what Australian philosopher and ecofeminist Val Plumwood calls Earthothers (2003), given our predatory ways and lack of value for animal and plant life? Our desire to care for, live with and respect Earthothers has become more acute as many more humans now suffer from the damage that we humans have wrecked on the environment. The impact of human habitat, extractivist practices and destruction on animal and plant life and the landscape in general has reached ecocidal extremes. The conundrum of how to care for more-than-human life is a theme running throughout the book.

Care for our life-worlds is full of conundrums. In recent years I have been learning about feminist political ecology and decolonial feminism as ways to shift the focus on the individual which is at the heart of the modern colonial gaze to see humans as belonging to communities and nature. I have had to consider how much I am personally and politically implicated as a white settler Australian now living in Europe, given the messy and violent histories of European domination that have erased other cultures and ways of being in processes of othering and hierarchical relations. Over the years I have had many guides that have helped me to shift my understanding of colonialism, neoliberal capitalism, racialised inequalities, interspecies and interethnic belongings in different life-worlds. I introduce some of those guides to you in the book. In the following vignette I share a story from my birthplace, Adelaide, about how important it is to be open to reappropriate, reconstruct and reinvent personal and political life-worlds.

The First nations people, the Kaurna, called the area around Adelaide *Tarntanya* (red kangaroo place). Before British colonial settlement in 1836, it was an open grassy plain with patches of trees and shrubs, the result of generations of land management. The River Torrens that runs through Adelaide was called *Karrawirra Pari* (red gum forest river) and provided water, fish and other foods. The colonial records state that the Kaurna people died from disease or were removed from *Tarntanya*. In the 1850s white settlers created the Botanical Gardens and the green parklands which today surround the city.

It is difficult to reconstruct histories of those early encounters in South Australia because white settler records conflict with the oral history of the Kaurna. One narrative speaks of peaceful settlement in unoccupied lands, the other of frontier conflict, introduced killer diseases and violent displacement. These are the 'narrative battlegrounds' between the documented and imagined history of white settlement and the Aboriginal oral history of the frontier. The historical and environmental damage continues to be embodied in collective memories.

On the Internet there is a photo of the 'last' of the Kaurna people, a woman called *Ivaritji* who died in 1931. Her eyes are haunting. But in revised histories she is no longer considered the last of the Kaurna people. Beginning in the 1980s, the histories of the Kaurna people have been reclaimed based on culture, place and language. *Nunga* has emerged as a general term used by South Australia for Indigenous Aboriginal people and a group of people speak for the Adelaide Plains and identify as Kaurna. Their reemergence reminds us that the history of white colonialism is tiny, even if hugely violent and destructive. Deep Indigenous cultural memories shift the white settler story when we recognise life-worlds based on millennial long histories and connectedness of people, plants, the animals and stars.

The conundrums of recognising different life-worlds means learning about individual, social, perceptual and practical experiences across time, space and body. It means being open to hope rather than despair and to look for new relations of care and possibilities of being-in-place and being-in-networks with other human and more-than-human beings. These are troubling and difficult conversations to which I return throughout the book, uncertain as I am of my positioning in these narratives.

In Chapter 3 I explore the concepts of Earthothers and Earthcare looking at living environmentalisms, ecofeminism and queer ecology. Among my inspirations are ecofeminist Val Plumwood, Vandana Shiva and Maria Mies, feminist political ecologist Giovanna Di Chiro and feminist queer ecologist Catriona Sandilands.

Vignette Three: Kinning

In 2023 I went to an exhibition entitled 'Metamorphosis' by the Australian artist Patricia Piccinini, her first show in The Netherlands. I have followed Piccinini's work for a while. She explores in eerily more-than-human sculptures the themes of love and care provoking us to ask questions about how technology, human beings and nature can co-exist in harmony. She explores the intrusiveness of technology and science on humans and more-than-human relations.[1] Piccinini's art draws out the viewers' empathy for her strange hybrid humanoid creatures shown in caring and loving positions. She destabilises our human focused, stereotypical imaginary around those we care for and are cared by. She poses questions about how humans relate to non-human others. Piccinini has worked with the renowned feminist science and technology studies scholar Donna Haraway, who also asks us to consider relationships with more-than-human others in equally provocative ways.

Haraway's call to 'make kin not babies' caused a small storm in the feminist world when it hit the academic press in 2015. She argued that we should 'find ways to celebrate low birth rates and personal, intimate decisions to make flourishing and generous lives (including innovating enduring kin – kinnovating) without making more babies urgently and especially, but not only, in wealthy high-consumption and misery-exporting regions, nations, communities, families, and social classes' (Haraway 2015: 164).

Like Piccinini's visual art, but in words, Haraway uses speculative fiction to consider how human and other-than-humans can live as kin. I find the idea of kinning with mountains, lakes, animals and plants unsettling. It is hard enough to relate and sustain ourselves and our human families or kin. How in our individual capitalist worlds can we see ourselves as members of multispecies communities? As one of the people living in a high consumption part of the world, should I now feel ashamed of having children?

There are several conundrums in this concept of kinning proposed by Haraway. And while I enjoy Piccinini's hybrid fantasy worlds, I am not sure of techno-hybrid futures or how to respond to the almost but not human care and love she depicts. The phrase 'making kin not babies' gets under my skin. It seems a hard call, especially given the joy I have with my daughters. I feel a sharp sadness when I hear young people questioning if they should have children as they consider the devastating impacts of climate change. As a feminist I fought for the choice to become a parent, technologically, socially and economically. I now see that such a 'choice' is deeply entangled in social and environmental collective responsibilities.

I have tentatively begun to pay attention to my relationship with different Earthothers in the environments that support and sustain me. Whether they are the oceans in Australia or the lakes in Italy or the woods in the Netherlands or the plants and flowers that grow on my terrace, I recognise I care for and feel joy in these living beings.

In Chapter 4 I go deeper into the concept of kinning, looking at the conundrums around populationism and choices to have babies, inspired particularly by Betsy Hartmann, Jade Sasser and Kalpana Wilson.

Vignette Four: Caring for the more-than-human

During my engagement with the community at the *Convento* in Bolsena, there were several tensions around running a crumbling monastery in rural Italy. Throughout the time I was engaged in the collective we struggled for funds to keep up the physical structure of the monastery. Energy went into everyday concerns of how to clean, fix the plumbing and care for the large garden. Even if the Franciscan order gave us usufructuary rights, a major headache was how to raise enough money to pay property taxes.

The daily business of taking care of family, an ancient building and the visitors required energy. We spent time figuring out who takes care of the people visiting the monastery and what happens with our families, when we were taking care of the monastery guests and the monastery itself. It was difficult to live an alternative life as a collective when we had to care for separate families under the shadow of the uncertainties of the Italian economic and political system.

Added to this was the issue of caring for the animals – the horses, chickens, goats, cats and dogs as well as the garden – the vines and olives, the soils and vegetables, particularly in the heat of summer. The collective became unstuck because we could not agree on the way to unknot our bodies, ecologies, technologies and times. The 'unexpected consequences of the stuff we don't want but must somehow accommodate' led to the group splitting (Piccinini 2006, quoted in Haraway 2011).

In recent years I have been struck by how many of my students speak of their care of plants. One PhD student filled her tiny house with plants seeded from her grandmother's garden thousands of kilometres away. She gifted me five of them and they now inhabit my windowsill, nestling together like a small jungle. She is not the only student who has asked me to care for loved houseplants when they leave the university. My small apartment is host to a crowd of plants, some towering over furniture, others being replaced over time as the winters take their toll. In turn, I ask others to care for them in my absence. One of my PhDs is now exploring plants as beings in the Netherlands, and we discuss the many plant connections in our lives. I confess to her I am guilty of enjoying the plentiful cut flowers which can be purchased for very little in the Netherlands. I have bought many roses that are flown across the oceans from Kenya to be sold in Dutch flower shops. They continue to grace my apartment in huge bouquets of dried flowers in second-hand copper and brass containers. They remind me of my grandmothers' love of dried flowers and the times I helped her arrange colourful Australian native flowers mixed with faded purple Scottish thistles we had gathered in the bush and fields near her beach house. Caring for plants and flowers are complicated emotional transactions.

In Chapter 5 I look further at these conundrums of care across species inspired by Maria Puig de la Bellacasa, Catriona Sandilands, Anna Tsing, Giovanna Di Chiro, Sophie Chao and Alexis Pauline Gumbs among others.

Vignette Five: Building communities of care

I was born in Australia with its complex and violent cultural heritage, and I then moved to make homes in different European countries with jobs involving travelling frequently over the years to attend international development forums. Not surprisingly, my sense of who I am has shifted in profound ways. Such intercultural weavings of self are not always comfortable, even if I have been consistent in what I cared about: justice, health, sexual freedom, gender equality and the environment. In my feminist advocacy and networking around gender and environmental issues, I had to learn not to impose on others my expectations of how and who and what to care about based on my class, education and whiteness, particularly in spaces that required a multiplicity of voices. Caring across difference has marked many of my personal and political friendships in transnational feminist and development spaces. My conundrum about how to relate and act with care about Global North/South relations, including Australia's deep-seated racism, seem to have increased over the years as I see the layers of power dynamics which are experienced as deeply personal as well as entangled in political, economic and social institutions.

I make sense of the world via an embodied sense of individuality, but also in terms of belonging to a community as I make connections with people and places as I have engaged in feminist and environmental politics. From my experience in transnational politics, communities are formed through meshworks, where people come together for an event and then may or may not meet again. Let me explain what I mean through the vignette.

My first engagement in European gender and development advocacy was when I joined Network Women in Development Europe (WIDE).[2] It was the base for my foray into transnational feminist advocacy in the 1990s, where we joined with other women's networks to lobby for feminist issues in the decade of the global United Nations conferences. We pushed for women's empowerment and gender equality, reproductive health and rights, sustainable development and human rights to be put on the international development agenda. With the (failed) promise of a peace dividend at the end of the Cold War in 1989, it was an invigorating time in which civil society and NGOs emerged as players in the UN development arena. But by the 2000s, many feminists were disillusioned with the depoliticising of the feminist agenda in the UN and were gathering around the World Social Forum (WSF), an alternative global meeting space for social and environmental movements and community organisations that did not wish to follow a UN-led agenda. I was invited together with another WIDE representative from Poland to attend the Feminist Dialogues of the seventh WSF held in Nairobi in 2007. WIDE was invited to represent all the Global North even if we were only a European network. The other twenty-three women who attended came from networks in Southeast and South Asia, Anglophone, Francophone and Lusophone Africa, Central and Latin America, and were representing the Global South. The confined voice of the Global North at the table was partly a deliberate reversal of the unequal representation of most global events, where representation of the North customarily overshadowed that of the South. It was also a signal that WIDE could be trusted in this transnational context to be in dialogue with the feminists from the Global South. In the dialogues we shared stories of women's concerns around increasing racialised economic inequalities, lack of reproductive and sexual rights, expropriation of social and environmental resources and erasure of Indigenous knowledge. WIDE was there to learn and listen to the Global South views and consider our responsibility and relationality with these women from their perspectives, not from our Eurocentric positioning. It was important that women from the Global North would give space to others rather than dominate the conversation or assume that the Global North experience of feminism was universal. Our dialogues included discussing the strategy to make feminist demands known in the other WSF events, via the media services and at the big plenaries which were dominated by well-known men. In the process a Feminist Dialogue text was agreed by the group, and we discussed who would deliver it and who would be on the platform. It was decided that white women from the Global North could be present on the stage, but they could not speak for the group. It was an important moment learning allyship and strategic presence. Behind the public scenes there were joyful times of sharing food, dancing and deepening friendships. The person with whom I shared a room I am still in close contact with, but upfront WIDE was the present, but silent, partner.

In such performances there is a strategic meshing of people and energies, but after the event the connections often unravel, and people move on. There is no expectation of continued organising. It will be in different permutations that people meet again. This loose process of meshworking is different from organised networks with management committees and different again from smaller communities, such as the *Convento*, either place-based or virtual, which endure over time as they build together with common purpose. I have belonged to these diverse types of communities since the early 1980s. They have been crucial politically and personally for my sense of well-being. They end or go dormant, but it is in these communities of care where I have found my vital energy and sense of purpose.

This freedom to organise and ability to commit struck me forcibly when my proposal to build a community of feminist scholars was awarded a large EU grant,[3] creating the possibility for research and networking among universities in several different countries. But there was immediately a conundrum of care because with the generous funding came a range of institutional demands, from using logos to complex rules on how the money could be used, a rigid governance procedure and compulsory extensive reporting. Over the five years the imposed governance mechanisms chafed at the feminist intent of the project. Academic institutional hierarchies and funding requirements flew in the face of what type of research could be done, and unsettled how the individuals in the network could relate and build community together. My personal conundrum was that when writing the proposal, I had placed intergenerational care at the centre, but in practice funding, institutional demands and competing geopolitical and generational dynamics wore down the good intentions.

In Chapter 6 I reflect on this conundrum by exploring what type of radical care enables communities to flourish, examining other forms of community building processes, looking at degrowth, commoning and community economies. I examine notions of radical care postdevelopment, degrowth, commoning and community economies inspired by feminist theorists such as Manuela Zechner, J.K. Gibson-Graham, Kelly Dombroski and Neera Singh.

Vignette 6: Care in the classroom

The last vignette reflects on the conundrums of teaching with care based on my reflections of a post-graduate Course 'The Making of Development', which I led for six years. I used post-development as a pedagogical tool. I was course leader with a collaborative teaching team made up of academics and MA students. We presented development as a highly contested term and we were honest in our doubts about the success of development processes. We pointed to the conflicts, contradictions and potential cracks in development theory and practice. We presented ourselves as co-producers of knowledge in the classroom together with the students. In the first year I taught the course some students met my pedagogical approach with disbelief, followed by demands to provide the facts and figures and the 'real development' story. The tools they wanted were not critical theory but practical information about how to do development better back home in their governments, NGOs and businesses so they and their country could benefit. But others saw what we were trying to do. To quote from one student who wrote to me with his/her reflection on the course:

> I want to thank you for the risks you take… You take a risk because of your teaching method. You take a risk when you let everybody express their own opinion, not knowing who is on the other side. You take a big risk with every single class you teach…. Given your status, you could easily rest and take no risks at all. You could teach in an 'ordinary' way. It wouldn't be the same for you, I am sure, but you could do it and nobody would demand you to change it. So, thank you for being 'extraordinary'. Please, keep taking risks. Now more than ever. You can't imagine how students treasure the professors willing to take the kind of risks you take.
>
> Student evaluation ISS, 2015

For me teaching development studies has been about taking risks to disrupt dominant narratives and open spaces. To paraphrase Paolo Freire, I see education as the practice of freedom to deal critically and creatively with reality and learn how to participate in the transformation of our world. Taking risks means you care for students' futures, even if at times such risk taking is not always immediately appreciated by students.

In Chapter 7 I conclude the book by pointing to the cracks and fissures in dominant development discourses and how to engage in encounters with different life-worlds; form connections among communities; understand human relations with Earthothers; and link academic discourse to processes of political change. I am inspired by scholars who engage with care in critical development studies and write about their pedagogical approach, from bell hooks' 'teaching to transgress' to members of the Cost Action 'decolonizing development' led by Julia Schoneberg and Lata Narayanaswamy.

Section Three: *Meaning making*

In the first two sections of this chapter, I have shared in a narrative style my personal/political experiences that led me to write a book about conundrums of care. In this last section I explain my methodological approach, which follows the tradition of feminist and environmental humanities of knowledge making through narrative writing, analysis, reflection and speculation.

My aim is to engage the reader with why the meanings of care I describe are embodied, experienced, evolve, relate, are many and complex, and are at times contradictory, hence the term conundrums. In this approach I take inspiration from Joan Tronto, who sees care as interwoven in 'our bodies, ourselves, and our environment' in a 'complex, life-sustaining web' (Tronto 2017: 31). I am also following Maria Puig de la Bellacasa (2017), who sees care as including everything and everybody, from the invisible care work of mothers, and those maintaining households, families, services and institutions. As I state earlier, care is the life-making and life-sustaining activities that maintain humans and more-than-humans that share our life-worlds. Understanding care means we embrace our multispecies relations with the earthworm as well as our entanglement with the modern technologies that dominate our landscapes. I am inspired by Puig de la Bellacasa and other feminist writers such as Donna Haraway (2016) and Anna Tsing (2015), who employ speculative fiction to analyse and imagine care otherwise. Thinking about care speculatively allows us to counter the erasures, invisibility and lack of value given to care by dominant power interests.

While I start from the human experience of bodies and human relations, I am speculatively looking to learn about care in relation to more-than-human others with attention to the material and physical processes that sustain ecosystems and human and more-than-human lives which make up our life-worlds. As Neera Singh states, all humans and more-than-human others are vulnerable and all are recipients and givers of care (Singh 2017). Understanding care requires us to address several layers of oppression such as the expropriation of women's bodies and social reproduction, racialised expropriation of peoples' and Earthothers' bodies and labours as well as colonial Indigenous and ecological dispossession. While acknowledging the huge scope of care as a factor in all our lives, at the same time it is important to see care in the context of various settings and from diverse perspectives in relation. I therefore give examples of care from both the Global South and Global North.[4] I pace the flow of the book by interweaving stories, both personal and speculative, with theoretical and conceptual discussions along with the examples of the practice of care from around the world.

Calling attention to the meanings and practice of care is a political project as we do so to make our collective worlds better (Puig de la Bellacasa, 2017). As Indigenous feminist scholar-activist Zoe Todd explains, 'reciprocity, love, accountability, and care are tools we will require to face uncertain futures and the end of worlds as we know them. Indeed, this ability to face the past, present, and future with care – tending to relationships between people, place, and stories – will be crucial as we face the challenges of these times' (Todd 2016: 383).

My analysis is necessarily situated and partial. I try to be as honest and transparent as possible about why I have selected these stories and certain writers, and give specific examples to illustrate conundrums of care. Care is one of the most debated topics in feminist theory. I point to some of the lively and crucial debates on care together in an accessible way that will explicate how care is understood in feminist economic debates on social reproduction analysis; interspecies relations in posthumanism; environmental justice in feminist political ecology; and is at the core of ideas of reciprocity and accountability in degrowth, community economies and postdevelopment/decolonial approaches.

Given the richness of these debates,[5] as with this introductory chapter, I open each chapter with a story designed to lead the reader easily into the chapter's themes. These narratives are personal reflections which point to the concepts and theories I want to explore in the chapter. In the other two sections of each chapter, I describe the concepts by highlighting the worker of the various writers I refer to above and by giving examples from different places, histories and cultures. I conclude with a short summary of the conundrums discussed in the chapter.

As I have pointed out in the Preface, I have taken the bold move to use storytelling to make sense of how I see the world and my place in it. This makes the book closer in its method to environmental humanities than social sciences. Stories help us to interpret reality through observation and sharing ideas: 'storytelling is theory and methodology, the vessel that helps us navigate diverse streams of knowledge, and the compass that orients us through the ebbs and flows of study and struggle' (Vasudevan et al. 2023: 1729). As black feminist theorist Sylvia Wynter (2003) has so powerfully told us, storytelling is what defines us as human. How we narrate our place in the world shapes our ways of knowing, being and acting, and transforms our bodies and worlds. Storytelling is an opening to the practice of imagining worlds otherwise.[6]

A note here on the possible conundrums of storytelling. I use stories to reveal the collective and political nature of personal experiences embedded in historical complexity, political struggle and difference. I embrace the critical potential in storytelling where 'stories recount particular experiences as rooted in and part of an encompassing cultural, material, and political world that extends beyond the local' (Fernandes, 2017, 4). However, in the development context storytelling has been undercut by scholars, consultants and political strategists who emphasise individual feeling, emotions and individual circumstances, disconnecting these stories from collective experience and macro structural power dynamics. As Sujatha Fernandes in her book *Curated stories: the uses and misuses of storytelling* (2017) states, there is now a strong neoliberal 'political economy of storytelling' (ibid., 10), where stories about pain and suffering of victims are produced to fit the strategic and measurable goals of development projects. In her critique of the US State Department and a women's storytelling project in Afghanistan she argues that storytelling of 'victims' is part of 'imperialist interventions', and in its consumption by western women's organisations, a continuation of 'colonial feminism' (ibid., 39). She calls not for sound bites and web profiles the reproduce structures of power, but for 'critical, complex, and contextualized storytelling that interrogates its material and historical conditions' (ibid., 66). Following Fernandes' critique of the storytelling that 'reproduce[s] global hierarchies and structures of power' as evidenced in development reports, I write transformative stories that consider the ways in which gendered subjects are produced, conscious of my own historical and political situatedness.

In Chapter 2 on 'Care Work', the opening story reflects on the Covid-19 pandemic and what we learnt about care as gendered, racialised invisible work. The second section examines care in social reproduction analysis in the paid care sector, as well as in the private sphere of families and interpersonal relationships, with reference to writers from the majority world. The third section shares insights into how different feminist projects are trying to revalue care in economics based on feminist policy and activist practice.

Chapter 3 on 'Earthcare' picks up the debates in Chapter 2 as it goes deeper into environmental justice, referring to ecofeminism and feminist political ecology's focus on care, looking at the critiques and concerns of assumptions about women as 'naturally' more caring. The chapter's opening story explores how famous narratives of Earthcare practices such as the historical Indian Chipko movement and the Kenyan Greenbelt movement continue to inspire environmental justice movements. The second section reflects on the insights of ecofeminists and critical Indigenous scholars through the concept of Earthcare, which helps to us to see human connection with the world of animals, plants and minerals. The section explores reciprocity and our responsibility with the natural world, learning from Indigenous writers as well as the tensions and possibilities for a reciprocal process of care, learning from First Nations' understanding of relationalities among peoples, places and Earthothers in our increasingly fragile environments.

Chapter 4 looks at 'Caring about having babies', asking who makes choices about if, when or how someone bears (or does not bear) children? Having babies – or not – is a deeply political question. The chapter delves into the heated global scientific and popular debates around the population, gender and environmental nexus which have divided feminists. We look at the conundrums that feminists raise as they share why they care about having babies in the face of climate change, and the recent debates in feminism, science and technology studies raging around the issue of population and environment.

Chapter 5 examines 'Interspecies Care' pushing further into nature/culture relations, with a look at how care is understood in the growing focus of humanities and social sciences on the interdependency of relations among humans and other species. The chapter's opening story reflects on changing attitudes to care for animals living with human families. The second section looks at wider issues around human relations with the more-than-human, looking at how human lives are entangled in the degraded landscapes we have shaped, oblivious often to the needs of other living beings. The third section looks at the complex histories of racism, power differences, subversion and loss through stories of care from environmental humanities, black feminist ecology and queer ecology.

Chapter 6 on 'Caring communities' focuses on scholars and activists in both the Global North and Global South who are analysing and building alternatives to mainstream development practices through postdevelopment practices, such as degrowth and community economies. The chapter's opening story recalls different experiences of building communities of learning and care in communities and social movements. The second section looks at the inspiring work of the community economies network following the approach of J.K. Gibson-Graham. It discusses the importance of ethical negotiations around everyday care practices and care when transforming economic practices at the community level. The discussion includes the importance of commoning and the collectivisation of care in conversation with degrowth. The third section looks at radical care and the support it offers to marginalised individuals, communities and life-worlds.

Chapter 7, 'Connecting with Care', concludes the book by bringing the insights from the earlier chapters to consider what paying attention to care means for critical development in theory and practice. The chapter's opening story takes up a story of my engaged connections with students, now friends. The second section reviews the conundrums of teaching development looking at examples of my own and other teaching practices emerging from places of radical vulnerability, hope and differential belonging, encouraging students to reimagine and repair our life-worlds. The third section looks at how development discourse needs to connect much more deeply to care as expounded in the book. It concludes the book by proposing a relational co-existence centred on care so that development can move towards just, sustainable futures, based on recognition of human and more-than-human agency.

Conundrums of caring conversations

In the book I use the word conundrum to refer to intricate problems that are difficult to deal with and do not appear to have obvious solutions. As care is an elastic concept, the book includes a wide range of conversations about the conundrums of care that touch a variety of difficulties. Such conversations stretch from the embodied and intimate to the abstract and global. The conversations relate to gendered bodies, specific places, diverse ecologies and alternative development proposals. The conversations are about the conundrums of how to provide care for children and older people as well as how to consider human responsibilities to care for other species. Most of all in the face of increasing economic and social inequalities, racism, conflict, environmental damage and climate crisis, we vitally need to consider how to practice care. This last is a conundrum that requires us to 'stay with the trouble' (Haraway 2016: 4). This is what this book aims to do – to turn difficult and caring conversations about collective experiences and knowledges into flourishing ways to build life-worlds for all living beings.

2

Care Work: Valuing Social Reproduction

The impact of the virus has exposed many weaknesses and vulnerabilities in modern societies ... care has 'come out', emerging from the shadows as a taken-for-granted afterthought in public life.
Michael Vine and Joan Tronto 2022: 202.

What we explore in this chapter

The Covid-19 pandemic put a spotlight on paid and unpaid care work of women – whether as nurses, domestic workers, mothers or daughters. Care work happens in all societies: children need to be looked after, homes need to be cleaned, meals have to be made, older people or those who are ill or disabled require constant care. These tasks are both onerous and rewarding whether the care work is carried out as a family member or a paid worker. Such daily jobs happen in the intimate spaces of our lives. These are what feminists in the Marxist tradition call social reproduction, and learning from feminist theorists and activists from the Global South, we can see these processes of social reproduction as 'life making' rather than 'profit making' (Mezzadri et al., 2025: 3). As we endured lockdown, Covid-19 underlined that it is care work which keeps our lives going. In this chapter we explore care work, not from an economic or legal perspective but from a feminist analysis of the conundrum that despite the massive importance of care work, it is still mostly invisible in the political sphere and undervalued in the economic sphere. I first look at the impact of the Covid-19 pandemic and what we learnt about care as gendered, racialised, undervalued and underpaid work. In section two, I present two vignettes of the complex interpersonal relationships of families and communities caught up in global and community care work. In the third section, I look at feminist care manifestos that emerged during Covid-19 in a strident call for a major revaluing of care.

Section One: *Pandemic crisis stories*

The impact of the Covid-19 pandemic varied according to where and with whom you lived and what work you did. If you were a legal citizen living in a small, well-serviced apartment in a European city with a salaried job, you could stay home and work online, have conversations via Zoom and binge watch Netflix. This was not possible if you were, for example, a migrant worker in an Indian city separated from family living in a rural village. There was no transport to travel home, no steady source of income and no access to the communication technologies which those living in the Global North took for granted. The pandemic situation underlined how much it mattered which state(s) governed your lives, which resources you could access, including basic food, water, shelter and health care. The impact of Covid-19 forced the world to appreciate and understand the importance of care work, paid and unpaid. The pandemic revealed the complexity of care work, made visible the care deficits, and reinforced a collective responsibility for care, the need to expand circles of solidarity and the lines separating 'us' from 'them'. The breakdown of families, the loneliness of the older people, and the deterioration of mental health, even in richer countries, revealed the importance of care as emotional and affective labour.

As Michale Vine and Joan Tronto (2022) note, the 'pressure cooker' of the Covid-19 pandemic opened up discussions on all aspects of care as many existing models, practices and assumptions proved inappropriate and the political dimensions of care became starkly apparent. Reflecting on the experience of Covid-19 they ask: 'How can care become part of the achievement of a more just world, rather than a casualty of its injustices? Can we use the opportunity to make matters of care, both large and small, more central to how we allocate values and resources, as individuals, as societies and as a global community?' (Vine and Tronto 2022: 305).

In considering these questions, I am inspired by Elke Krasny's 2022 monograph on feminist responses to Covid-19 and her invitation to see feminist worry and hope as a way to revalue care and our visceral connections with others, including, even, the air we breathe.[1] As Krasny writes:

> The Covid-19 pandemic was a global lesson of care in breathing and shared air.... Breathing is not a choice.... Breathing is a matter of life and death. Breathing, at the most fundamental level, connects humans with one another and with the planet as a whole in interdependency and vulnerability.... Protecting others from one's own breath and protecting oneself from the breath of others, in order to avoid infection, became a global task and responsibility.
>
> Krasny 2022:20

At the onset of the pandemic, March 2020, I was in Uruguay. I had to rush back to Europe before airports closed, arriving at Schiphol on the last flight. I had spent several hours before boarding in Montevideo trying to find masks. For the next two years masks were a feature of all our lives. As Covid-19 is still with us, I keep a stack in my hallway. Covid-19 has made us aware of breathing, virus transmission and our embodied connections with others. At the height of Covid-19 we became aware of where it was safe to breathe, with whom we could share the air, where infection might come from. Our relations to our bodies changed. I became acutely aware of my chronological age, what my body – clocking in at late fifties – could sustain. I found it touching but dismaying that students would offer to shop for me. I became aware I was protected and cocooned in privilege. When vaccinations became available, I was in European countries that made them freely available, and I was high on the list to receive them and had the wherewithal to access them. Covid-19 made me breathe, see, feel and experience care in different ways.

The hardest experience for me was that my 90-year-old father became ill and died during Covid-19 in Sydney, Australia. Studies have shown how isolation of older people during Covid-19 led to physical and mental deterioration (Lithander et al., 2020). My father was a gregarious man who thrived on contact with others. Being weeks at a time isolated in a hospital ward with no visitors, not even my mother, and unable to use a mobile phone, he visibly shrank and then died.

As an Australian citizen I was able to go and visit him when the country had closed its international borders. I was required to stay in a quarantine hotel for fifteen days, even though there were no cases of Covid-19 in Sydney when I arrived. It was a comfortable hotel, with a view of Darling Harbour from generously sized but permanently shut windows. During those fifteen days I had face to face interaction with people only twice – two fully masked and gowned nurses who appeared at the doorway for one minute to take a Covid-19 test. Food was delivered in paper bags outside the room, and we were told there were police stationed at the end of the corridor to ensure you did not escape from the hotel.

To offset panic and claustrophobia I learnt to breathe slowly and deeply by doing online yoga and meditation. I would watch TV and the mounting figures of death and illnesses from Europe and other parts of the world. I would worry I might be carrying the virus, feeling concerned and guilty at the responsibility of whether unknowingly I might infect my father, and, it seemed, the whole of Australia. Meanwhile I kept breathing in my closed hotel room.

Once out and proven Covid-19 free, I was reunited with my father. His smile made it all worthwhile. I took deep breaths relishing the familiar scent of Australian eucalyptus. At night I slept outside on my brother's verandah off Tamarama beach listening to the waves, watching the stars and breathing in the fresh night air.

My personal story is intermixed at a distance with far more tragic stories of the millions who died during the pandemic and the restrictions and oppression so many experienced. Following Krazny, I too worry that Covid-19 revealed 'how deeply human beings have failed in ethical and social terms, to develop a culture of care for living together with their planet' (Krazny 2022: 22), and like her, I write in the hope it is not too late.

Whether Covid-19 opened a portal of possibility or not,[2] it did kindle feminist hope that care work would be revalued given the visible increase in women's care responsibilities due to the pandemic and the failure of states to respond (Blanco and Cuervo 2021). The physical and mental health of those involved in caring labours were neglected, put under huge stress and in many cases, risks and danger. Women across the world worked much longer hours at home than men, taking care of those around them. Globally women suffered increased domestic abuse and violence, including emotional violence. The pandemic exposed the 'essentiality of care, the structural and pre-existing crisis of care' including the need for 'planetary care' (Krazny 2022: 123).

Since Covid-19 we are learning to breathe, learning to care in new ways, aware of our multispecies interconnectedness and interdependency in the face of humanity's careless ruination of the planet. To again echo Krasny, we have had to learn to live in an infected world. Revaluing care is one way to start.

Section Two: *Valuing care work*

In the recent decades there has been a lot of writing by various feminist theorists, particularly feminist economists, to make care work visible and valued.[3] The pandemic was like a magnifying glass; it made existing gender, race and class inequalities worse. Despite all the banging of saucepans in appreciation of doctors and nurses in 2020, the figures reveal the gendered dimensions of increased formal and informal care work for women in homes and communities during Covid-19 (Agarwal 2021; Kabeer et al. 2021; DAWN 2022; Harcourt 2023). There is a strong social bias that does not accord value to the care work that (mostly) women do, either for free or for poor wages in private homes, hospitals and in the community.

There are several conundrums to consider here. One is that women do care work because they care about others. It is part of the feminine role women are socialised into taking up care as their expected duty. Caring is part of a feminine identity. Women, it is assumed, join the paid care work sector because they are (naturally) caring and can (naturally) help others. So, the logic goes, they do not need to be paid well, because women already feel innately rewarded by doing the caring, therefore, they do not need to be further rewarded by receiving good work conditions or wages. So, care work, even when paid, is not rewarded fairly. Care workers meet other people's needs as part of their relationship. It is a mix of duty and love (Fisher and Tronto 1990; Folbre 2014).

The second conundrum is that even if care workers 'do not need' to be paid well, because they are considered unskilled and ultimately doing what women 'naturally' do, nevertheless there is a huge profit to be made by the market and the state in paid care services for childcare and older people. Particularly with patterns of ageing shifting and the increasing needs of older people in the Global North (and among the rich in the Global South), care is a growing sector for investment that sells care at a vast profit, taking advantage of the low wages paid as the care work itself is not valued (Folbre 2017).

A third conundrum is that although care work is integral to being a good mother, wife, daughter et cetera, there is also a strong class and race component as to who does the care work. Richer women, to free themselves for other tasks, pay other women to do care work. Domestic paid care work is done largely by poor and racialised women. The paid care sector exploits women of colour and migrant workers. This is a global pattern across different welfare regimes. Studies of the global care chain (a metaphor that suggests care is something that is shackling people together as a necessary burden) show how in the Global North, the ageing population and the increasing numbers of people living beyond working age leads to a huge care deficit where rich countries do not have enough workers to do the necessary care jobs (Budlender 2010, Banks 2020, Folbre 2017, Fraser 2016). This paid care sector, despite the deficit, is marked by low pay and poor working conditions as care markets are becoming globalised to meet the needs of those located in richer global locations, while those in poorer locations scramble to meet their own care needs (Tronto 2010). Women from the Global South or poorer parts of countries move to Global North countries or to larger towns or cities to do those jobs. Many of these workers are overqualified, undertaking transnational parenting and doing poorly paid care work, which is nevertheless physically demanding, mentally and emotionally stressful. Undocumented care workers are the most vulnerable, treated as disposable, unprotected labour. As the pandemic showed, care work is not an inexhaustible resource. People cannot provide good care when overworked, tired without job security and experiencing a lack of dignity and a sense of self-worth. It leads to high levels of burnout where people are weighed down by repetition, meeting the unending needs of others (Murphy 2015; Curty 2020, Rai 2024).

Feminists write about the politics of care looking at how global capital is extracting care, primarily from women, to maintain the social context for economic production (Ojeda et al. 2022: 163). As Nancy Fraser famously stated, 'the economy free rides' on care work which she describes as the 'activities of provisioning, caregiving, and interaction that produce and maintain social bonds' but which are accorded 'no monetised value' and treated 'as if they were free' (Fraser 2016: np).

Shirin Rai in her book *Depletion* (2024) examines the human costs of caring across class, race, gender and generation. With examples across the world she shows how care work when unrecognised erodes lives, families, communities, societies and ecologies. For her the conundrum is that instead of care being a joyful practice it is draining, a depletion. She looks at how the growing cost of care and caring for our social and ecological worlds is leading to depletion and calls for 'strategies for recognizing, measuring, pluralizing, and reversing the harms of depletion . . . in the context of the growing costs of care and caring for our social and ecological worlds' (Rai 2024: 18).

A last set of conundrums around care work is set out in an article by a group of Marxist-feminists (Mezzadri et al. 2025), which reflects on what the Covid-19 crisis meant for the concept of social reproduction, considering the gendered and racialised experiences of care, labour and exploitation in the Global South. In their reflections they warn 'of Anglo-American supremacy, Eurocentrism, and epistemic violence' and the need to challenge 'the Global North epistemological privilege' (ibid.). Gender theorising is not free from 'histories of colonialism, racial capitalism, planetary migrations and planetary crises' (ibid., 6). They call for feminist analysis to challenge Global North ideologies and for 'plural understandings of social reproduction' and concepts like 'care, community, affection, solidarity, and emotional labour' (ibid., 7). Such a plural approach would mean recognising that 'housing precarity and insecurity, experiences of the cost-of-living crisis, experiences of unpaid/underpaid care labour, anticipation/fear of future unmet care needs, and experiences of community activism' (ibid.,8) have to be embedded within the structural changes in the political and social relations that govern the world.

The conundrum here is how to build solidarities among different locations while at the same time challenging historically Global North-centric universalisms. In revaluing care it is important to recognise the plurality of feminist insights of experiences of social reproduction as life-making in different contexts. While finding ways to acknowledge distinct experiences and histories of marginalisation within diverse locations, it is also important to bring these knowledges together to revalue care work in broader political, economic and social transformation.

To puzzle out further the conundrum of care and how to give social, economic and political value to care work, I now turn to two vignettes building from different meanings of care work from the experience of migrant care workers in Italy and community organising of care in Chile and Spain.

Vignette One: Is a migrant care worker 'one of the family'?

Alexandra is an Italian working mother in her late thirties, with three children under the age of 10 living in a comfortable home in a large Italian city. Rosa is a Filipina care worker in her early forties who is employed by Alexandra.[4] Rosa has two teenage children, who are living with their father and grandmother, Rosa's 60-year-old mother, on the island of Mindanao. Rosa sends money regularly to the family and is hoping to bring her oldest child over to Italy. She keeps in close contact with her family via What'sApp and since moving to Italy ten years ago, she has returned to the Philippines twice.

Rosa lives with Alexandra and their family in a small bedroom with her own bathroom near to where the three children sleep. She does most of the household chores, including preparing meals and cleaning the house. She is given public holidays, one evening and Sunday off a week. She has an employment contract, which means she is accumulating a pension. Her pay is a comfortable 1,000 Euro a month with board, which is above the going rate. In the last few years, she has also helped Alexandra to manage a second apartment as an Airbnb. She often accompanies the family on holidays.

Rosa speaks of the opportunities she has been given and how good her conditions are compared to other domestic care workers in the city.[5] Rosa misses her family but considers the community around her Church, whom she meets regularly, to be an important social support. Her aim is to provide the opportunity for her children to come to Italy and expects that Alexandra and her husband would be the sponsors and support her family reunion.

Alexandra considers Rosa one of the family and is particularly appreciative of her help for the Airbnb, which brings in money to supplement Alexandra's consultancy work. After five years, Alexandra feels they have settled into a pattern which suits Alexandra's work and the family's needs well. Alexandra feels she looks out for Rosa and offers her the best conditions she can. She is not sure about sponsorship for Rosa's children, as that would mean Rosa could not live-in.

During Covid-19 Rosa was in lockdown with Alexandra and the family. Alexandra did the home-schooling and Rosa the domestic tasks. Rosa worked longer hours, and did not have time off, but was grateful for the security during difficult times. She spoke of other domestic workers who were not living-in who lost their jobs and their income. Covid-19 reinforced the idea that Rosa was one of the family and was expected to take up more tasks with no increase in pay.

This vignette shows a good working relationship where a paid care worker living with a family is valued as one of the family, at least in the employer's eyes. It is evident that Alexandra is the employer who is determining how Rosa is contributing to the family's care. Rosa's own interests – how to keep a close connection with her family in the Philippines and church life – are not considered part of the relationship for which Alexandra is paying. There is a maternalistic attitude towards Rosa, which is emotionally complex, but also a way to keep control of what she does as a care worker, leading to long hours and demands; for example running the Airbnb, babysitting after hours in the evening and coming on holidays primarily to take care of the children. On the other hand, the shared everyday lives lead to intimacy and closeness in the caring for children and the shared home space. The conditions of work and emotional commitment to the other woman's needs are negotiated unevenly between the employer and employee across socio-economic, cultural and racial divides.

You could argue that the maternalism Alexandra is exhibiting is itself a form of care (Marchetti 2016). Alexandra considers she is providing and protecting Rosa and welcoming Rosa into the family. Beyond the generous pay, Alexandra considers she is providing access to the family's social network and comfortable way of life (the family own two holiday houses by the sea). Rosa, in return, expresses a strong sense of moral indebtedness and gratitude. This is not an uncommon situation; the name for this type of gratitude among the Filipino community in Italy is *utang na loob* (Banfi 2008: 151).

Rosa is part of the Filipino diaspora – a transnational workforce of migrant workers in Italy who are providing care in domestic homes and in hospitals and care homes (Marchetti 2016; Banfi 2008; Magat 2004). They care not only for children but the growing number of older people who need 24-hour assistance. Middle class families prefer live-in help by a reliable migrant care worker to placing their older relatives in poorly run public care homes attached to hospitals or religious institutions. In Italy there is not yet a plethora of comfortable well run expensive private care homes, as in other Western countries. In 2022 there were 14 million people in Italy over 65 years of age.[6] Care for elder people is largely undertaken at home with the so-called 'migrant-in-the-family' model. Where once family, primarily daughters and wives, were responsible for providing care, now over a million foreign workers (those that are documented; there are many more illegal care workers) have replaced or supplemented family members as live-in or day carers for the estimated 2.8 million older people who require care.[7] Most people expect to be cared for at home, even if not by a relative. For example, there is an insurance offered by Allianz in Italy that would pay for monthly live-in help to avoid moving to a public care home, and the government offers support to refurbish a home to enable a failing older relative to stay.

Filipino migrants have stepped in to support mostly middle-class families who pay for care and domestic tasks in homes as well as in the health sectors. The accepted narrative of these (usually) women's lives is of selfless, even heroic, migrants who support their families back home as they work long hours caring for other families/ people. Filipino migrants are seen as hard workers, able to have good relationships with employers and embedded in families who care – reinforcing a sense of how generous the employer is. This narrative ignores the long hours and actual sacrifices being made by the care workers (Banfi 2008: 164). As in the case of Alexandra and Rosa, there is a blur between paid and unpaid work. Rosa is relatively lucky, as she has the required documents, through the support of Alexandra (who agreed to sponsor her and to navigate the Italian bureaucratic system). Other domestic workers staying for equally long periods might not get the same support and fail to get the documents. But even with the documents and permission to stay, which allow them to acquire citizenship, workers like Rosa are considered at best partial citizens (Banfi 2008: 153).

In this maternalistic setting, where Alexandra 'generously' helps Rosa, who is grateful for her job, the kindness and comfortable housing plays down that this is a contractual arrangement. The employer's willingness to help, for example Rosa counting on Alexandra and her husband to sponsor her children, is seen as a benefit, not a right, one that depends on Alexandra, not Rosa. As Sabrina Marchetti points out, maternalism, though making life comfortable, reduces Rosa's possibility to ask for her rights as an employee (Marchetti 2017).

Such working conditions for migrant domestic workers in Italy reflect a care order based on global care chains (Ehrenreich and Hochschild 2003; Yeates 2004 and 2009; Todaro and Arriagada 2020), where it is the norm for migrant workers to do the work that Italian women once did as their familial duty, or that poorer women carried out for other Italian families for little pay. Such a system does nothing to uphold the rights to care, but has a created a system which expects migrant women to be the people who gratefully provide care work in Italy, while their own families benefit economically but suffer in other ways.

The conundrum is that Filipinas like Rosa are content to be in this situation as the closeness and friendship makes life away from family and home bearable. Being a dutiful and trustworthy worker means that employers provide care workers with access to a variety of benefits. In the literature Filipinos are reported as seeing this highly personal and interdependent relationship as positive and a good working arrangement (Basa et al. 2012; Magat 2004; Marchetti 2017). Issues like rights to a liveable wage leading to a liveable pension are not on the table, so that even if they are doing essential labour, once they grow older they will not have an adequate income to stay in Italy. The issue of transnational families and the problems of children growing up without their mothers, husbands and wives, not living together for many years, are hidden beneath the apparently cosy maternalism.

Vignette Two: Making visible care work in community organising

In the first vignette the focus is on interpersonal relations rather than collective political engagement of care workers. The majority of the invisible care workers are not engaged in making change but try to make the best of what their individual situation offers. The second vignette is about how care workers have come together collectively to challenge their situation at the political level. I move from my anecdotal reflection on maternalism to two examples of community organising and demands for a revaluing and recognition of care work. I look at two such examples, one in Chile and the other in Spain.

The first example comes courtesy of my work in an international development studies institute, where I have the privilege of learning about care work from young scholars who have gone on to build care work policies after returning to their country. I have written elsewhere about one of my students (Harcourt 2023) who after writing her MA thesis on parental leave and care penalties in Argentina (Cirmi Obon 2017), returned home to become National Director of Care Policies in the newly created Ministry of Women, Gender and Diversity, to support reform of the care system in Argentina. Sadly, the Ministry was immediately dismantled with the change of government in 2023, reminding us of the transitory nature of politics and the fickle possibilities for transformation relying on state policy.

Another ISS MA student wrote her thesis on contested care politics during the Chilean referendum on changing the constitution in 2022, in which revaluing care work was one of the reforms proposed. She analysed how fourteen organisations formed a coalition to push for care as the axis for the new constitution. Despite the failure to establish a new constitution in September 2022, she argues that the process led to a greater visibility of feminist visions of care and that feminist care politics were now in dialogue with state policy.

I have continued to be involved in her study of community care in Chile. We have explored how the voice and concerns of care workers have been integrated into a new care policy that aims to address the undervaluing and inequalities of care work, and care provisioning (Bravo Arias 2022).[8] We argue there is a reframing of the care system in

Chile, where the knowledge and experience of care workers are being recognised in social protection policies. Covid-19 drew attention to the importance of the public provision of care in marginalised communities when community care networks provided care in remote areas where few state services were available or could reach the population. Policies are now proposed that promote economic autonomy for care givers within the family as well as domestic care workers. For example, some state and local authorities plan to provide training, tele-assistance, better care centres and monetary compensation through decent work legislation.

This result came from intensive lobbying by feminist organisations working with care worker organisations, including the research of the feminist network *Carpa de las Mujeres*, who in 2021 mapped out how care work operates in different communities. Their mapping showed how community care functions with few resources filling the gaps left by the state. It mapped out how care work for children, older people and people with disabilities is largely carried out by women inside families, through unpaid care work or by poorly paid migrant women care workers from rural areas or nearby countries such as Peru.

Bravo Arias (2022) documents how such care workers have become more vocal about their vital role in providing care as they have joined feminist organisations to fight for their rights as caregivers, mobilising for greater responsibility of the state on the provision of care. In these demands care workers are not the objects of concern, but rather are voices in the debate with their knowledge and labour part of the feminist political discussion.

The rights of care workers are currently being integrated into policy design for a reformed care system in Chile. The reform process has included community-led dialogues organised by the Ministry of Family and Social Development (MDSF) in 2023 involving 12,000 people, the majority of whom were care workers. The engagement of care workers and feminists in policy reform in Chile is a vibrant example of the rising visibility of the politics of care in Latin America, which is revaluing care in a process in which care workers are the subjects rather than the objects of policy.

While this is an important example of how care feminism is influencing state policy, there remains the conundrum of whether by engaging in advocacy and policy for pay and infrastructure, care workers are intrinsically losing how to organically care within the community. Increasing state and local policy around care could lead to unwanted scrutiny in the home as standards could be applied that might reinforce dominant (for example medical) understandings of how to do care, failing to acknowledge diverse approaches to giving care that might be harder to measure or monitor. While it is important to reward and recognise care giving and care work, there is a danger that certain forms of care are not seen as appropriate according to standards that are set outside the community. There could be the risk that what might then be perceived as non-conforming caring is treated punitively. Or it could become that only through pay to individuals or certified organisations is care work valued, rather than building stronger bonds through collective care for others that responds to community needs as they emerge.

Moving away from demands for fairer pay and better policy I turn to the second example in Barcelona, Spain and more radical ways of understanding care. The vignette is based on the inspirational research of Manuela Zechner (2015, 2020, 2021).[9] Like Krasny, Zechner writes with passion and hope about care as central to radical transformation. Her descriptions of caring communities in Barcelona illustrate how unpaid care work can be seen as an act of solidarity in clinics, neighbourhood networks and collective childcare. Care work in this context is understood as self-organised support and help for each other in everyday lives, building on peoples' collective needs and desires rather than determined by the market economy.

Zechner has written extensively about radical collective care, sharing her activist engagement and her research with new municipalist movements in Spain, specifically Barcelona *En Comú*.[10] She describes the politics of neighbourhood childcare in the political and social landscape of Barcelona between 2016–20. Her focus is on how mothers – women, migrants who were mostly informal workers – came together in the urban context of Barcelona in a variety of actions to reconfigure care for children and pregnant women, ill and older people and people with disabilities. The actions range from strikes and demonstrations to public debates to democratise care and envisage care as best practised when seen as a commoning of resources. She calls this 'municipal politics from below'. The role of care is part of the politics of the Spanish feminist movement's challenge to models that privilege wage labour over unpaid work and reframe citizenship to include care.[11]

Zechner was involved in networks of mothers organising childcare who sought to make childcare visible in political organising and organisations, so that care for children becomes part of the shared responsibility of the community. She describes how childcare is built into the activities of networks of mothers who take care of each other, as well as children, working together to find resilient and sustainable places and practices where care for others is valued not in market terms, but in terms of belonging and cooperation. In these networks care work is not mediated by market or state. Instead care work is shared collectively and cooperatively so that the wider organic benefits are felt by all. Mothers exchange advice, gifts of food and other objects, take joint walks, facilitate playdates, organise workshops and campaigns, and circulate information ranging from the medical to the political and the personal. They learn about ways to build sustainable alternatives to the public and private nursery systems for bringing up children and creating community.

These concrete experiences of childcare common in Barcelona are an example of care feminism and a radical politics of care in the Global North. They differ from the example of Chile, where the focus is on demanding pay and thereby formal recognition of care as work by the state and market, and are very different from the Italian example of one end of the global care chain, which is marked by maternalism. Instead Zechner's research in Barcelona is about mothers in communities organising care as a commons practice. It is about solidarity and collective actions that centre care as part of the politics of place, which define stronger bonds and commitment to one another. The conundrum here is that this is materially possible because Barcelona is in the Global North, where there is more accessible wealth and possibility, and reflects a particular culture searching for alternatives to individualism. Nevertheless, how such radical communities find resilience and sustain themselves depends on state systems which give access to functioning infrastructure, schools, hospitals, roads, sewerage, running water et cetera. Access to which is much more sporadically available and, in some places, unattainable in the Global South. The time that can be taken to devote to childcare work depends on public structures functioning well, and the fact that there is enough wealth circulating to allow for organising, workshops, playdates, walks et cetera. So, while inspired by such endeavours it is important to consider the context. How to create the time and space to care is, as Tronto states, 'among the most important considerations in rethinking society from a caring perspective' (2013: 166).

These two vignettes from Chile and Barcelona show what rethinking care could mean in terms of revaluing care work, understanding relations of care and feminist strategies of collective care. At the heart of these vignettes is how to revalue relations of care in homes, communities and policy. What the stories show is that revaluing care is not only about monetary value but changing how we see care as vital to a good quality of life, recognise the time needed for it, respect those who are performing care, and acknowledge the labour and skills that go into care work and the considerable political effort to change care policy and practice (Zechner 2021; Mezzardi 2022; Barca 2024).

Section Three: *Feminist recovery plans and manifestos*

A feminist politics of care is not only about putting monetary or market value on care work, but it is also about creating a deep systemic change so that care work is understood to be at the heart of sustaining life. During Covid-19 when care work became visible and labelled as vital work, many innovative feminist recovery plans emerged that pushed for more systemic change (Krasny 2022: 111). I now turn to some of these manifestos, which present strong feminist imaginaries of how to care differently at a systemic level. These manifestos are aimed at international and state institutions, and propose not only how to recover from Covid-19 but also how to avoid returning to business as usual. Leaving aside the question of how far the policy process did change, and to what effect, what is important about these manifestos is that they brought together policy makers, public administrators and researchers together with feminist grassroots organisations, activists and civil society groups to consider how to revalue care work (Krasny 2022: 131). The statements show what feminism learnt from the catastrophe of the Covid-19 pandemic as well as the looming climate crisis. In the following section I look at their proposals for change in a review of feminist recovery plans and manifestos for better care politics and economies of care.[12]

The *Hawai'i Feminist Recovery Plan* 2020 of the Hawaii State Commission on the Status of Women[13] challenged the Hawaiian state to change the focus of public sectors and services and support land- and sea-based practices traditional to Hawai'i's ecological and food system. The *Hawai'i Feminist Recovery Plan* focuses on the importance of caregiving associated with and expected of women in marginalised racial, Indigenous and economic groups. The plan brings the knowledge of marginalised women to address the crises in healthcare, social, ecological and economic policies exposed by the epidemic. Learning from this community, the recovery plan speaks not only about response and recovery, but also of 'repair and revival: repair of historic harms and intergenerational trauma playing out as male domination, gender-based violence, economic insecurity, poor health and mass incarceration. These are a serious threat to a sustainable, resilient society. It is clearer than ever that capitalism could not care for us during COVID-19' (*Hawai'i Feminist Recovery Plan* 2020: 1).

The plan sets out how to revive 'place-based practices and knowledge, and self-determination that enables our connections, inseparably economic and social, with women, one another, and with the wider world in order to build bridges to a feminist future for Hawai'i' (ibid., 4). It underlines the need for a deep cultural change which focuses on relations of care to reverse climate change, repair historical violence and inequality within and between countries, address inequalities within households and value 'all members of the communities beyond their value to economic production in capitalism' (ibid.,17).

Reflecting on the impact of Covid-19 in the UK, *The Care Manifesto. The Politics of Interdependence*, written jointly by The Care Collective (Andreas Chatzidakis, Jamie Hakim, Jo Littler, Catherine Rottenberg and Lynne Segal) argues forcibly that the pandemic dramatically exposed the violence of neoliberal markets and the incapability of caring for people even within homes, illustrating the 'unbearable collective anxieties of living in an uncaring world' (Care Collective 2021: 4), and where 'neoliberal economic growth policies have become dominant in so many countries, the inherently careless practice of "growing the economy" has taken priority over ensuring the well-being of citizens' (ibid., 8).

In response to the violence and lack of care during the Covid-19 period, the Manifesto argues for a 'politics that puts care front and centre' (ibid., 5). They define 'care' as nurturing welfare and flourishing: 'Care is our individual and common ability to provide the political, social, material, and emotional conditions that allow the vast majority of people and living creatures on this planet to thrive – along with the planet itself' (ibid.,7).

The Manifesto lists ways to begin to address 'the pervasiveness of carelessness' by building on the examples of 'care-inpractice' (ibid.,19). Care-inpractice examples such as communities supporting older people, neighbours sharing home grown food, setting up swap shops and skills sharing workshops, and volunteer groups caring for animals and forest life illustrate mutual interspecies interdependencies and the intrinsic value of all living creatures as part of a grassroots place-based political mobilisation (ibid., 22).

The Feminist Recovery Plan Project of the University of Warwick (Natile 2022)[14] also envisages the Covid-19 crisis as an opportunity to reimagine the policies by placing grassroots activism at the centre of policy. The project's plan sets out to build on feminist grassroots activism to place social reproduction at the centre of socio-economic-legal systems and the environmental and climate crisis. Activism is understood as an important form of social reproduction work, invisible and unvalued but necessary to bring about social change.

At the international level, The Global Alliance for Care, which was publicly launched by the National Institute of Women in Mexico in alliance with UN Women in December 2021, sets out why a focus on care is crucial to avoid crises. *Beyond Covid-19. A Feminist Plan for Sustainability and Social Justice* (2021)[15] presents to policy makers the key levers to catalyse a green and gender equitable recovery. Through different financial, management, governance and knowledge mechanisms the plan aims to put in place gender-just transitions which will support women's organisations and protect female human rights defenders. The documents assembled in support of the plan map out transformative policies on livelihoods, care and the environment.

These manifestos and plans are examples of feminists envisaging new caring relations. They point to how care work enables communities to flourish. They address policy and politics to strengthen care work practices among communities that were made visible as vital work during Covid-19, building on grassroots community care work and activism. They are developed with historical awareness of structural injustice and hope for the end of economic and political exploitation of care.[16]

The first conundrum is that while these plans and manifestos are important statements, did they lead to change? While we remain hopeful that they succeed, it is not yet evident that there is a new global care order in the making. Even if they prove unrealistic in the short term, I would argue that they offer important ways to think about care work as part of our collective resilience and ability to find ways to live sustainably. We should not lose sight of what they propose, particularly given that the disruption caused by the pandemic, political instability and climate change is set to continue. It remains a conundrum that if these propositions were to be taken up, they would change the way the economy and polity function. Paying attention to care work means we would need to slow down and adjust to complex, messy and not always predictable ways of living. Our current world is dominated by speed and innovation that assumes there is progress that can be measured. There seems to be no time to care. Care is antithetical to dominant images of modern economic living. Centring the care work of the marginalised and oppressed, the unseen and unmentioned is profoundly radical as it draws attention to why we need to challenge dominant imaginaries of boundless horizons of economic growth that are built on the lack of care of others, indeed on carelessness. Tronto calls this dominant form of care wealth care (caring for wealth not people). She points out how wealth care shapes our political economy so that we principally care for wealth (and celebrate the obscenely wealthy 1%) in such a way that profit and economic growth are the central activities and purpose of society. Such wealth care leads to both the extremes of wealth and poverty, as well as to the exploitation of nature (Tronto 2023).

Conundrums of care work

In contrast to wealth care, the examples in this chapter centre care work in social, political and economic life. They show how care work requires time, skill and knowledge, and support. Moving towards a world where care work is visible at the centre of our economy and polity means recognising that we are all interdependent on care, even if care work differs according to the context, requirements and needs for care shift over time.

The Italian vignette points to the racialised and gender exploitation of migrant labour that has global dimensions. It reflects a care order based on global care chains where it is the norm for migrant workers to do the work Italian women once did as their familial duty or poorer women carried out for other Italian families for little pay. Such a system is not based on the rights of those who do the care. Although the Italian system relies on migrant workers, if they manage to get papers to stay they are not considered true citizens. The conundrum of transnational families and the problems of children growing up without their mothers, and husbands and wives not living together for many years, are not visible in the Italian State, which has accepted the migrant-in-the-home model without providing security or rights for the migrants. Another conundrum is the intimacy and sense of being part of the family that is created, often leading to relationships based on maternalism, where Italian women see themselves as offering support and opportunity to care workers living in close proximity, failing to see the exploitative nature of the relationship.

The chapter also points to how recovery from catastrophes like Covid-19 needs time, imagination and change. The feminist manifestos and plans call for radical political change so that care work responsibilities are a substantive part of democratic life. Such a political agenda is about care for humanity and also for the planet (Arora et al. 2020). Imaginaries of care and new politics of care not only ask that we refuse wealth care, but extend our understanding of care beyond rights for humanity to the rights and care of and with the planet. In the next chapter we look at the concept of Earthcare and how feminist and other writers call for care for and with the world of animals, plants, oceans and minerals.

3

Earthcare: Ecofeminist and Indigenous Approaches to Our Life-worlds

If our species does not survive the ecological crisis, it will probably be due to our failure . . . to work out new ways to live with the earth, to rework ourselves. . . We will go onwards in a different mode of humanity, or not at all.

Val Plumwood 2007: 1.

What we explore in this chapter

In this chapter we go deeper into environmental justice, looking at the insights of ecofeminists, feminist political ecologists and critical Indigenous scholars as we explore the concept of Earthcare and the human connection with the world of animals, plants, oceans and minerals. After sharing three personal encounters with Earthcare in section one, in the second section I explore the concept of Earthothers guided by Val Plumwood and Deborah Bird Rose, and in the third section I reflect on what we can learn about responsibility and reciprocal relations from the intercultural weavings of Indigenous scholars.

Section One: *Stories of Earthcare*

I first experienced what Earthcare meant when I attended the Miami Congress Women for a Healthy Planet in November 1991. The event brought together over 1,000 eager and committed women from around the world. Far from being a soft or romantic idea, I learnt Earthcare was a feisty and politically demanding practice. The Miami conference was full of women speaking about their campaigns to combat environment devastation, end colonial and military conflict. They were boiling with political rage and radical hope. The Congress remains one of the most thrilling international conferences I have attended (and I admit to attending quite a few). It opened with an acknowledgement of the tribal lands on which we were meeting led by Indigenous women of the Tequesta tribe. This was the first time I had witnessed a ceremonial honouring of First Nation's people and their land at an international event. There were daily tribunals with statements of powerful Women's Justices from around the world. All participants joined regional caucuses to contribute their views to the final conference statement. It was heady stuff. The meeting was orchestrated by Women Environment and Development Organization (WEDO), an international non-government organisation led by former US congresswoman Bella Abzug, who at seventy years old was still a firebrand.[1] The passionate and heartfelt discussions were inspired by stories told by grassroots women leaders from around the world. The Congress collectively produced a dynamic manifesto called the Women's Action Agenda, which was defiantly anti-colonial, anti-military and anti-neoliberal economic development. In this outspoken agenda Earthcare was about solidarity, action and demanding space for women's voices to be heard to care for the planet. Women spoke about their responsibility to care, but they were not prepared to be the ones who cleaned up the mess given they were excluded from the institutions which created the mess in the first place. As Abzug stated: 'Women do not want to be mainstreamed into a polluted stream. We want to clean the stream and transform it into a fresh and flowing body. One that moves in a new direction – a world at peace, that respects human rights for all, renders economic justice and provides a sound and healthy environment' (Dankelman 2010 quoting Abzug at the Gender CC Women for Climate Justice Panel 2009).

The Congress participants met in one of the huge edifices of glass that make up Miami city, a massive urban development that had erased the 'river of grass', the Everglades. It served to highlight a major conundrum given the purpose of the Congress. The extensive ecosystem had been cared for by the Tequesta peoples for thousands of years but was destroyed when the land was exposed to colonial and economic exploitation draining the rivers and wetlands, severely damaging the ecosystem in the nineteenth century. This eco-crime was spelt out by the US journalist and environmental activist Marjorie Stoneman Douglas, then 100 years old at the Congress (she lived to 108), when she spoke about her decades of collective struggle to preserve the Everglades. She embodied a powerful example of the fight to care for the Earth against the destructive power of extractive agricultural and business interests.

Although organised by Abzug and her New York-based team, it was the women from the Global South who the Congress acknowledged as the leaders in global women's critique and action for a healthy planet. Their testimonies spoke of the power of Global South women's leadership in caring for the Earth with courage and determination. I felt history was being made as I sat in the enthused audience listening to women such as the winners of the Right Livelihood Award,[2] Wangari Maathai and Vandana Shiva.

Vandana Shiva's now classic ecofeminist book *Staying alive* (1988) had brought to the world's attention the rural women Chipko movement's non-violent resistance to save trees from commercial logging and deforestation in the 1970s. Clad in a vivid colourful sari, her testimony in Miami argued that women had to resist the maldevelopment of science and economic development. She underlined that in their struggles against patriarchy, rural women were a source of crucial insights and vision.[3] The tall and majestic Wangari Maathai (who later went on to become the first African woman to win the Nobel Peace Prize in 2004) testified how the Green Belt Movement mobilised Kenyan women to plant more than 30 million trees through tree-planting campaigns selling seedlings for reforestation.

The powerful narratives of Earthcare that so resonated with me in Miami have continued in the narratives and actions of women's movements, writers and scholars I have encountered over thirty odd years, including those relations forged in the WEGO network.

Among such encounters in the WEGO network was with feminist activist Seema Kulkarni. In January 2020, I met her in person in Maharashtra when I visited a WEGO PhD student she was hosting.[4] I was greeted with kindness by Seema and her team, who immediately invited me to join them in a hot spicy meal of local delicacies. When Seema and others saw my reddening face and gasps for water my meals from then on were confined to rice, plain vegetables and tea. This thoughtfulness (and the embodied nature of difference) is indicative of how well I was cared for in my visits in and around Pune to meet small holder women farmers, where I caught a glimpse of the profound work Seema was doing with different organisations.

Seema is a founding member of the Society for Promoting Participative Eco-system Management, Pune (SOPPECOM), where she coordinates activities on gender and land, water and sanitation and is the National Facilitation Team member of Mahila Kisan Adhikar Manch (MAKAAM) Forum for women farmers' rights. MAKAAM is a nationwide alliance of farming women, women farmers' collectives, civil society organisations, researchers and activists. Their focus is to support small holder women farmers' access to land and livelihoods as well as to acknowledge their important care work for the Earth, their families and communities. As Seema describes it, Earthcare is the fight 'to rebuild our soils and our lives through agroecological farming. . . reimagining our world that was in harmony with nature while addressing discrimination based on class, caste and gender' (Barca et al. 2023). In this framing Earthcare is closely linked to demands for social justice. Following Maria Mies (1998), Seema advocates not only to give value to women's unpaid care work in the household and other non-wage subsistence work, but also to acknowledge the work of nature and her regenerative cycles.

In a more recent encounter in 2023 I found myself cycling through the rain to an early drinks party held in an unfamiliar part of The Hague. Establishing my bearings, with a glass of wine to hand in the rapidly filling room, by chance I introduced myself to Farah Obaidullah as 'Wendy, an Australian working in The Hague'. Farah however recognised me from a talk I had given some time back, and we were able to make a real connection over our concerns for gender and environment. Farah is founder of 'Oceans are Us'. She cares passionately about the fight for healthy oceans, which she sees as fundamental to the wellbeing of all living beings. She campaigns for greater awareness of the impact of climate change on oceans, the dangers of overfishing and the looming threat of deep-sea mining. Her concern is palpable at the loss of global wildlife and natural systems. She sees deep-sea mining as a critical threat to the oceans which make up 70% of our planet, arguing it will cause irreversible damage to the deep ocean, disturbing locked-away carbon and destroying life. As her website states: 'The High Seas belong to all of us. Rather than start a new era of colonialism, laying claim to the treasures of the deep, we must designate the deep-sea a sanctuary for peace and science! Join me in being a voice for the ocean.'[5]

Speaking to her in conversations since, I realise how caring for the earth extends to the seas and changing our use of them as massive waste sinks, and unlimited supplies of food. Instead, we need to build awareness of care for the oceans as part of Earthcare. Farah is a member of the network 'Women4Oceans', a group of women who work with coastal communities and oceans for better planetary and human health. They, like Farah, care that the voice of the ocean is heard.

In the book she edited, *The oceans and us* (2023), Farah brings to our attention the women who are caring for the ocean. They elaborate the 'dynamic, fluid and interdependent relationship we have with the ocean' (Britton 2023: 297). They describe what is happening to the oceans due to climate change and the devastating impact of humanity on seascapes and the creatures that live within them. They underline humanity's emotional connection to the ocean. The book gives practical suggestions for how, as part of citizenship science, we can help to clean up the ocean, record sightings of marine life or report sewerage flows and other human waste that is threatening the sea and our life with it (ibid., 304). The book details reciprocal care of the oceans and humanity countering the stereotypical masculine image of the hardy sea farer conquering the ocean. Instead, the book presents the ocean as a global commons that requires respect and care. The book illustrates how local communities around the world practice care for the ocean as a global commons, including women scientists who tend not to be professionally recognised (Giakoumi et al. 2021).

I share these stories about a tiny fraction of Earth carers, to underline the conundrum that even as such women keep the world alive through their knowledge and actions, they are invisible in the 'mainstream narratives of the catastrophic earth-system change epoch that scientists have called the Anthropocene' (Barca et al. 2023). Earthcare needs to be seen as integral to an on-going reproduction of earth systems or the historical relations of care between humanity and nature. Stefania Barca (2020) calls this 'forces of reproduction', which expresses itself in political struggles at global, national and local scales. Such embodied knowledge and experience need to compliment or perhaps counter the dominant narratives of political ecology. Barca describes the forces of reproduction as the Earthcare labour of tending to the soil, water, animals, plants, that are 'part of the web of interdependencies which keep people alive'. For Barca, Earthcare is 'the production of life' (Barca 2020). Earth carers make us aware that we need to act with responsibility and to care about relations. They create spaces where resistances to dominant narratives can be cultivated, and radical possibilities exist. They shape strategies for environmental justice based on alliances that work towards a liveable future based on their knowledge that can repair and regenerate our planet. Their actions and stories point to hope for a world different from the one we currently inhabit; if we can learn, unlearn and relearn about what Earthcare requires to restore our rapidly deteriorating life-worlds.

Section Two: *Earthothers*

While I started this chapter with my personal encounters with Earthcarers, my understanding of their importance is deepened by writings of academic feminists from different disciplines and places. These academic reflections show the importance of cross-cultural understandings of human and more-than-human wellbeing as we rethink our most basic narratives about how humans can live in relation to animals, plants, minerals, soil, wind and sea.

A major influence in my understanding of Earthcare is the late Australian ecofeminist philosopher Val Plumwood, who coined the term Earthothers to animate our relations with all the other beings that inhabit our world. The term Earthothers helps us to understand that that other beings such as animals and plants should be seen as persons and that our human lives are lived in relationship with these other persons (Plumwood 2003). In her writings (and life) Plumwood asks us to build new forms of ethical practice amongst human and more-than-human subjects learning from past, present and future, where care is seen as a core to safeguard planetary wellbeing.[6] She helps us to consider what needs to be redressed in our multispecies relations as we renew responsibilities for the life-worlds we inhabit.

Plumwood critiques anthropocentrism using radical ecosophy (Plumwood 2003) in ways that show we relate to humans and Earthothers not just with our rational mind but also with our emotions, bodies and hearts. She undoes human exceptionalism insisting that we have to understand our relations as humans in the natural world, we are embodied, embedded in nature: 'ecologically embodied beings akin to rather than superior to other animals' (Plumwood 2008: 89). In other words, we need to situate our lives in ecological terms and see Earthothers in ethical terms.

Plumwood wrote a powerful story that I continually refer to in my teaching and writing: 'The eye of the crocodile' (2008), published posthumously, that illustrates this way of understanding humanity in relation to ecology, and the ethics of how to relate to Earthothers. In the story she narrates how in 1985 she was attacked by a crocodile while canoeing in Kakadu National Park during the season when crocodiles are territorial. She was taken into a death roll by the crocodile three times before escaping by scrambling up the riverbank. She uses this story to share her insights into animality, embodiment and relations of humanity with Earthothers as she ponders the idea of thinking flesh and knowing flesh. As she was rolled by the crocodile she had become part of the natural food chain. In reflecting on this harrowing experience, she reflects anew on ecological relations with the world where nature and animals are sentient beings and kin.

Learning from Plumwood we can see that humans are mutually dependent on Earthothers in entangled relationships of connectivity. We need to recognise our connection with Earthothers so that rather than trying to control and dominate them, we learn 'creature-languages of the Earth' (Rose 2013a). Instead of trashing Earthothers, destroying life through violence, we can forge different ethical practices founded on an awareness that humans exist together with Earthothers. This a vital realisation if we are to truly care for our increasingly fragile environment.

After her near-death experience with the crocodile, Plumwood proposes that 'our worldview denies the most basic feature of animal existence on planet earth – that we are food and that through death we nourish others. Death at the level of the ecological community, it can affirm an enduring, resilient cycle or process' (Plumwood, 2007: 67). In a later publication she writes, 'By understanding life as circulation .... We can learn to look for comfort and continuity, meaning and hope in the context of the earth community, ... to displace the hierarchical and exceptionalist cultural framework that so often defeats our efforts to adapt to the planet' (Plumwood, 2008: 101–102).

For her the body,

> does not just 'end' – it decays or decomposes, its matter losing its prior organisational form and taking on or being incorporated into new forms in a sharing of substance/life force. The recognition of life as in circulation and of our death as an opportunity for other life can discourage the human greediness ... privilege and technological mastery.
>
> Plumwood 2008: 105

Her profoundly philosophical insights about Earthothers and the Earth and our need to rethink our relations with them are made explicit in her powerful storytelling. She invites us to continue to create stories of our connection with Earthothers:

> We are in desperate need of stories that create much greater transparency of these relationships in our day-to-day lives. We must once again become a culture of stories ... This is the real meaning of ecological literacy ... we have eliminated the stories that connect the two realms [of nature and culture].
>
> Plumwood 2008: 44–45

In her stories she explores how care for nature and culture come together. In her essay 'Memorium to Birubi' she narrates her twelve-year long relationship with a rescued orphaned wombat, Birubi. She describes how he belonged to both the world of her house and that of the forest on Plumwood mountain, where she lived. Their relationship cuts 'across the usual boundary between the wild and domestic, the forest and the house, the non-human and the human, nature and culture' (Plumwood 2008: 51).

She shares their intimate and rich life together, where 'the great gulf of difference was part of the magic of the relationship'. She describes the 'privilege' to come to know a free and basically wild animal and the enchantment when they walked together along a forest track, and when she would look up from her desk to find a wombat sitting in her armchair by the fire.

She recognised in Birubi a strong sense of self and stubbornness which 'meant that you were dealing with a real other; that contact had to be on his terms and not just on yours' in contrast to domesticated animals like dogs. Her care for Birubi meant knowing he was 'wily, wary and tough', yet he allowed her to care for him. She felt his fear and his need for freedom, even if 'every time he left the house I knew that he might be badly injured or that I might never see him again' (Plumwood 2008: 55).

Plumwood's writings and life have left a strong legacy that echoes throughout ecofeminist writing and practice in Australia and worldwide. Stories of care and love surround her as she touched the lives of many. One moving tribute by her close friend and colleague Deborah Bird Rose tells the story of Plumwood's burial in 2008 on Plumwood Mountain, where she and Birubi had shared their twelve years together. Bird Rose describes how a large butterfly settled on Plumwood's body during the outdoor burial service before it disappeared into the forest. Bird Rose writes how those gathered there 'were awed by the connection between Val, the butterfly and the forest' and how 'This awesome moment was expressive of much of Val's philosophy. We saw before us the intentionality of other creatures – always mysterious, but never mindless – and we experienced ourselves as creatures who are attentive to others and who are participants in the life of the world' (Bird Rose 2013b: 93).

Deborah Bird Rose, an anthropologist, philosopher, storyteller and advocate for social and environmental justice, who lived for most of her adult life in Australia, also contributed inspiring writings on humanity's reciprocal relations with Earthothers. Her writings are embedded in her learnings from the communities *Yarralin* and *Lingarra* in Australia's Northern Territory. She writes of the violence of colonisation which encroached on lands oblivious of care of generations of people.

Her work exposes the effects of human actions on the nonhuman world highlighting the Indigenous sense of ecology as one of connectivity and mutual benefit in place. She acknowledges how she learnt from Indigenous teachers the importance of responsible relations – that human beings should not be 'in an extractive relation to "resources" but have a responsibility to ensure the abundance of all other life into the future' (Bird Rose 2024: 24).

She proposes that we learn to see how ecological systems are composed of conscious beings – humans and Earthothers – who communicate, act and react. As Bird Rose stated:

> My research with Aboriginal people in Australia has strengthened and deepened my understanding that life emerges from dialogue amongst persons; it depends on relationality, interdependence, and mutual flourishing. In this context, persons are mindful beings. And in contrast to western binaries that would put humans on one side of a boundary where mind and culture are pervasive, and put everything nonhuman on the other side of that boundary, asserting that there is no mind or culture over there, Australian Aboriginal people, like Indigenous people in many parts of the world, understand the world they live in to be saturated with mindfulness.
>
> Bird Rose 2013b: 6

This underlying vision unites human and nonhuman, body and spirit, ideal and real and future possibilities of flourishing in the face of anthropogenic disaster (Bird Rose 2024: 27). Bird Rose describes how she was aware and respectful of the ontological frictions between Indigenous and western views, an approach she named 'firestick wisdom' (Bird Rose 2024). White settlement and dispossession led to degradation and devastation, where 'cattle have caused the loss of water, with rivers receding and becoming shallower, and a host of edible plants diminishing or disappearing altogether – yams, seed-bearing plants and bulbs and parsley-like plants that grew around springs and billabongs. Bandicoots, bilbies, brush-tail possums and "native cats" have all disappeared' (Bird Rose 2024: 26).

In supporting First Nation's fight for reparations, she underlines how ecological devastation massacres and dispossession disrupted millennia of Indigenous Earthcare of Country. Her writings are dedicated to social and ecological justice as she bridges the gap between Aboriginal and settler Australians, situating her work squarely in a critical analysis of colonialism and genocide while at the same time arguing that life-worlds are always becoming (always emergent). Her work is in dialogue with Plumwood and also Indigenous thinkers such as Steve Meredith, Old Jimmy Manngaiyarri, Kathy Deveraux and others. Bird Rose, like Plumwood, sees the need to learn how to communicate with Earthothers, through creature-languages. She quotes Steve Meredith, Ngiyampaa Elder:

> They [experts] tend to look down and study nature, like it's ants on the ground. But when you fall asleep, eh, them ants they'll crawl all over you.
>
> Bird Rose 2003: 98–99

In her first book, *Wild dog dreaming* (2011), Bird Rose describes how dingoes (seen as pests by white settler farmers) were poisoned, dying painful deaths. For Bird Rose dingoes are beings, plants are sentient, and the Earth itself has culture and power within it. She sees (western) humanity as 'the species that is generating vast wreckage upon the lives of others'. She argued that the spirit is continuous after death. The dingoes continued to kill in afterlife, as living creatures fed on poisoned dingo bodies died, so that the poison moves through generations and across species lines. In a later essay Bird Rose reflects on her emotional outrage when witnessing the public display of dead dingoes. She describes as being 'haunted by dead bodies, living bodies, Dingo families (human and nonhuman), stories, teachings, and the beautiful harmonies that dingoes send out across the night air, and which here had been so suddenly and brutally cut off' (Bird Rose 2011: 10).

Seeing the death of dingoes demanded response: 'I write in between betrayal and recovery, between fast action and slow heartbreak, between quick outreach and deep experience... I write so that we of the living, even we who are lost and alone, can be called again into remembrance' (ibid.).

While sharing the pain and loss, she demands humans take responsibility. There are possibilities for change as the world is always emergent, and our decisions are part of the world's becoming. This sense of hope in the possibility of flourishing multispecies worlds in the face of growing destruction is captured in her last book: *Shimmering* (the third book in the *Dreaming Ecology* series, published posthumously in 2024). Shimmer *Bir'yun* is an Aboriginal aesthetic that helps call up multispecies worlds: 'the shimmer, the brilliance, and, the artists say, it is a kind of motion. Brilliance actually grabs you. Brilliance allows you, or brings you, into the experience of being part of a vibrant and vibrating world' (Bird Rose 2024: 53).

Bird Rose explores the 'matrix of power, desire, and lures and to move across several species and cultures to draw our attention to the brilliant shimmer of the biosphere and the terrible wreckage of life in this era that we are coming to refer to as the Anthropocene' (Bird Rose 2017: 51).

She narrates how a group of Earthcarers, volunteers and scientists, work together to protect flying foxes in peril. She describes that 'Flying fox carers are one set of passionate people who work at the edge of extinction and who have opened their lives and homes to others' (ibid., 52). She describes the caring of flying foxes as examples of 'beautiful modes of careful attention ... as relational responses that ... enable us to participate in the shimmer of life' (ibid., 60).

Flying foxes also shimmer as they carry seeds of trees on their fur, tongue and wings 'bringing the animal to the trees and bearing the trees' gifts along to other trees. At the same time, a new generation of flying foxes is nurtured into life with lashings of glorious nectar' (ibid., 59).

Her exuberant writing points to a conundrum that 'We are called to live within faith that there are patterns beyond our known patterns and that, in the midst of all that we do not know, we also gain knowledge. We are called to acknowledge that in the midst of all we cannot choose, we also make choices' (Bird Rose 2017: 61). Not knowing but living in hope that flourishing is possible, trusting in mystery, this helps us to survive the mourning and sadness for the world that is so damaged.

In her story about flying foxes in a world of peril she concludes: 'We are. . . called into gratitude for the fact that in the midst of terrible destruction, life finds ways to flourish, and that the shimmer of life does indeed include us' (Bird Rose 2017: 61).

Before moving onto the next section I need to pause and reflect on another conundrum that presents itself when I write about white settlers learning from First Nations peoples, particularly as I am a white settler Australian now living in Europe: how to ensure that we are not extracting knowledge and objectifying Indigenous people as we seek to understand their life-worlds. It is important to acknowledge that it is not possible to write as if that knowledge is separate from demands for reparation which are part of the continuous fight of First Nation's peoples to pursue claims for past and on-going colonial injustice, and to increase their personal freedoms and political autonomy. Bird Rose bridged different ways of seeing the world because of her long engagement with First Nations peoples, so her stories and reflections draw attention to and disrupt the damaging impact colonisation has had on Indigenous peoples and the intergenerational and cross-cultural transmission of their knowledge. By acknowledging the *Yarralin* mob as her teachers over the years, she calls attention to them as knowing subjects from whom she is learning. She challenges western ways of knowing and what constitutes knowing. As a writer and storyteller who lived relationally with First Nations peoples she exposes on-going practices of colonisation, and the past and present devastating impacts of the global world order on ecological systems. She helps us to see that our life-worlds are emergent, shaped by the relations among First Nations peoples, settlers and Earthothers. Such an approach underlines that 'Indigenous peoples exist in meaningful, substantive, embodied, powerful ways that are independent from the violence of colonisation' (Nakata and Maddison 2019: 419).[7]

These writings acknowledge the past and on-going violence that First Nations peoples face. They also honour and learn from Indigenous knowledge in respectful ways as part of the broader justice project to unsettle colonial indigenous-settler relations. In sharing how inspirational I find Plumwood and Bird Rose writing on Earthothers, even if I am only a conduit, I do so to encourage you to feel the depth of these two original and powerful writers' insights.

Section Three: *Intercultural weavings*

I acknowledge there is a conundrum in trying to learn from knowledge that is embodied in history and places that are read in profoundly different ways. I can only grasp the surface of what is possible to know about the land I was born as a white settler and from which I live far away now in Europe. I still, though, see the possibilities of learning from Indigenous peoples' understandings of reciprocal processes of care for Earthothers. My focus in this section of the chapter is to open ways to learn from writers from Indigenous cultures. Their work helps us to come closer to understanding Earthcare as a response-ability based on the reciprocal relations among peoples, places and Earthothers in our increasingly fragile environments. In their writings there is also the demand for reparations for the destruction of more-than-human beings through colonisation, extractive capitalism and global patterns of racism. I find these create troubling questions about care in response to violent resource extraction, extinction and the destruction of cultures resisting and healing colonial violence. Here I am interested in writings which help to define Earthcare in ways that thread together different knowledges and stories, helping us to co-create life-worlds.

I have been inspired by writings of a collective that co-write with Bawaka Country to acknowledge the importance of Caring with Country (the term used by First Nations Australians for human and more-than-human communities sharing land or place or landscape) and First Nations Australians' deep notions of care as human responsibility to live with and nourish, spiritually and physically, the beings that are part of Country.

Country is described as 'an integrated, more-than-human presence that incorporates land, animals and people, but also nonhuman beings such as tides, waters, winds, insects, rocks, plants, languages, emotions, songs and ancestors (Suchet-Pearson et al. 2013). Indigenous Australians' way of being with Country is founded in an 'ethics of collaboration and care, based on recognition of human and non-human agency, is one that would nurture relationships, responsibilities and accountabilities within and beyond the false dichotomies of researcher–researched, manager–managed' (ibid. 2013). In sharing their way of being with Country, we are invited to imagine ways to reworld and reconnect with each other to care for the

Earth by fostering cross-cultural understandings of human and more-than-human wellbeing.

'Caring for Country' encompasses 'looking after all the values, places, resources, stories, and cultural obligations associated with that area, as well as associated processes of spiritual renewal, connecting with ancestors, food provision, and maintaining kin relations' (Hill et al. 2013: 1). Care in this context is a complex relational practice which connects people to Country and to other forms of wellbeing including mind and emotions, body, family and kin, community, culture and spirituality. Country allows for a vibrant understanding of the interconnectivity of place and space where understanding Country is about caring for all humans and more-than-humans. It is important to understand there is no one understanding of Country, as understandings of Country have evolved over 65,000 years, including during the last centuries of violence and change. Knowledge comes from living with Country, 'learning (through hearing, feeling, doing) the language of its soils and winds and birds, and in becoming together' (Bawaka Country et al. 2016: 464). In an article Bawaka Country including Sandie Suchet-Pearson, Sarah Wright, Kate Lloyd and Laklak Burarrwanga (2013) explains the way Caring for Country is lived through their description of the gathering of miyapuna mapa (turtle eggs) as part of the Yolnu ontology of co-becoming.

> What it means to see humans as one small part of a broader cosmos populated by diverse beings and diverse ways of being, including animals, winds, dirt, sunsets, songs and troop carriers, we argue for a way of knowing/doing which recognises that 'things' can only come into 'being' through an ongoing process of be(com)ing together. They are never static, fixed, complete, but are continually emerging in an entangled togetherness. Fundamental to this ontology of co-becoming are key lessons around attention, responsibility and ethics.
>
> Suchet-Pearson et al. 2013: 186

In articles, talks and films,[8] the community living with Bawaka Country show how Indigenous peoples and local communities have profoundly challenged the dominance of industrial resource management regimes in a variety of ways over decades since white settlers came to Australia. Despite colonialism, First Nations people have continued to interact physically and spiritually with their Country and shaped their life-worlds and life ways. They call for all Australians to practice an ethics of collaboration and care, based on recognition of human and non-human agency, which nurtures relationships, responsibilities and accountabilities. They challenge the language of separation between human and nature, human centredness and control over nature and speak instead of mutuality, of connectedness, of becoming-together, respectfully and carefully. Rather than conserve, or develop, extract or own Country, they argue that humans need to communicate and act responsively as beings belonging to Country and pay due attention to the connections that bind and constitute them to a multitude of other sentient beings or Earthothers. Their stories invite all of us to consider our complex interdependence and mutual connection with nature, in whatever place we are living: 'all humans and non-humans, actors, actants, everything material, affective, all processes and relationships, are not *things*, are not even isolated *beings*, but are entangled becomings, creative and vital and always in the process of becoming through their connections' (Suchet-Pearson et al. 2013: 187). Such articles help us to understand Earthcare not only from an empirical social science standpoint but also with our emotions, bodies and hearts. Their writing is sonorous, reflecting the beauty of their thoughts.

In writing this chapter I frequently paused to reflect on the conundrum of how to learn across differences in conversations about Country/territory/Earthothers as a white settler Australian living in Europe. As I write I look out my windows at European landscapes that carry the tread of centuries of change through urbanisation, industrialisation and environmental degradation. It can be a strain to understand how to re-imagine ourselves ecologically and through connection with the world of animals, plants and minerals when Earthothers seem to be controlled totally by human need, from the tended gardens to the glass house vegetables and flowers, fields of wheat and animals in machine-run farms. Even the weeds in the cracks seem to be allowed temporary respite before they are chopped down. I feel at times heavy of heart to learn the language of Earthothers where there is such control, enmeshing ourselves knowledgeably into the creature-languages of the Earth means also to recognise the mess we are in.

Potawatomi Nation botanist Robin Wall Kimmerer[9] helps us to understand how we could live in reciprocal and ethical ways with Earthothers. As both an Indigenous and scientific scholar her work helps us to weave together peoples, places and Earthothers as we learn to care about our increasingly fragile environment. As a writer and a scientist, her interests in restoration include not only care to make ecologically aware communities but also care to learn old/new relationships with land. Kimmerer writes on plant ecology, traditional knowledge and restoration ecology. In reading her stories I feel hope in Kimmerer's statement that 'Language is our gift and our responsibility. I've come to think of writing as an act of reciprocity with the living land' (Kimmerer 2013: 347).

I listened online in November 2023 to a talk Kimmerer gave at Cornell University where she spoke about Indigenous wisdom, scientific knowledge and the teaching of plants. She wove together western and Indigenous knowledge as she explained the need for gratitude to and responsibility for Earthothers: 'Healing the damage of the Earth takes a powerful form of reciprocity, a powerful form of justice... We have had a feast, both given to us by the Earth and taken from the Earth. Now it's time to do the dishes' (My notes from Robin Wall Kimmerer, Lecture on 'Land Justice: Engaging Indigenous Knowledge for Land Care' at Cornell University, 1 November 2023).

Her focus is the restoration of lands on Turtle Island (North America) which have been damaged by resource extraction, habitat loss and toxic contamination. She invites us to consider an Indigenous world view: 'That we all share this habitat, that all of us should have a voice in how that land cared for and cares for itself' (ibid.). This requires that western science is in symbiosis with traditional ecological knowledge so that we do not separate empirical, rational observation from emotional and spiritual knowledge values. Kimmerer describes this as a 'two eye seeing' model, i.e., sustainability requires Indigenous science as well as western science. Indigenous caretakers know how to care for land using the tools of Indigenous science where ecological restoration is inseparable from cultural and spiritual restoration. Sustainable restoration draws upon people's knowledge and relationship with the land. It is as much about restoring relationship as it is about restoring damaged ecologies. It requires 'authentic ceremonies of gratitude, healing, and reconciliation between the people who wrecked that place and the place and the original caretakers' (ibid.). It requires decolonising the story of what is land, what is nature and what is human responsibility towards Earthothers.

Kimmerer's book *Braiding Sweet Grass* helps to decolonise the story. As she states in the Preface:

> This braid is woven from three strands: indigenous ways of knowing, scientific knowledge, and the story of an Anishinabekwe scientist trying to bring them together in service to what matters most. It is an intertwining of science, spirit, and story – old stories and new ones that can be medicine for our broken relationship with earth, a pharmacopoeia of healing stories that allow us to imagine a different relationship, in which people and land are good medicine for each other.
>
> Kimmerer 2013: x

When describing the 'Onondaga Nation Vision for a Clean Onondaga Lake' she describes the need to listen to the Earth and to be in a relationship with it. 'Nature herself is a moving target, especially in an era of rapid climate change. Species composition may change, but relationship endures. It is the most authentic facet of the restoration. Here is where our most challenging and most rewarding work lies, in restoring a relationship of respect, responsibility, and reciprocity. And love' (Kimmerer 2013: 336).

Earthcare means more than scientific ecological restoration; it means recognising that in healing the land, we are healing ourselves. Kimmerer gives us a strong sense of hope that we can learn reciprocity, so that 'as we work to heal the earth, the earth heals us' (Kimmerer 2013: 340). Learning from Kimmerer and other Indigenous scholars, Feminist Political Ecologists in their writing on Earthcare aim to 'open up space for recognizing, envisioning, and making life-affirming ecologies rather than extractive systems of destruction' in ways 'capable of protecting and defending life and living worlds' (Ojeda et al. 2022: 150). They place care issues at the centre of environmental critiques as a way to encourage reciprocal relationships among and between people and living beings as part of the growing concern to defend commons around the world that are sustaining life and are 'part of emancipatory emergent ecologies that are care-focused and life affirming' (ibid.,157 and 158). These hopeful framings of Earthcare are inspired by studying with movements such as the Zapatista Movement in Mexico, the Adivasi Land Rights movement in South Asia, or the Melanesian Land Defense Alliance in the South Pacific (ibid., 158).[10] These movements act with a strong sense of responsibility to care for the environment where nonhumans have their own agency, spirituality, knowledge and intelligence (Whyte 2018: 127). As J. K. Gibson-Graham stated, 'something else is caring for us and the earth, or contributing vitality to our complex co-being' (2011: 4). We have to recognise that everything is interconnected and look at how 'our solidarity' can extend to the more-than-human, and how we are connected 'to ecologies, to Country' and in this way 'usher in new forms of belonging' (ibid., 17).

Conundrums of Earthcare

I have proposed in this chapter that Earthcare requires learning from ecofeminism and Indigenous knowledge how to reflect on relationality and be in dialogue with Earthothers. Traditions built on intimate relations among people and Earthothers have been undermined by colonisation, capital extractivism and global expansion but their knowledge is not yet gone. Recognising the importance of Earthcare helps us to be open to other possible worlds so western scientific knowledge is twinned with other knowledges about nature-social relations. Being open to encounters with Earthcare takes us away from human exceptionalism and invites a different kind of politics, knowledge and way of living that is interconnected and co-constituted with Earthothers. As Cristina Yumie Aoki Inoue states: 'Indigenous ways of knowing and of being on the planet can contribute to understandings of Earth politics in the Anthropocene that stress humans' nonexceptionalism and all of the political relations that follow from such understandings' (2018: 33).

The conundrum is how to engage seriously with Earthcare and not dismiss it as fantasy, romantic, untenable in today's 'modern' world. There are many powerful economic and political competing interests around which ecologies are contested and negotiated. Can we reconstruct our understanding of our natural and social world from the perspective of the multiple cultural and ecological practices that continue to exist among Indigenous communities? These are serious epistemological, cultural and ecological questions.

This chapter, and book, are part of my journey of self-reflection and dialogue on how to learn and respect from ways of living with Earthothers. I am inspired by people who are weaving cultures together as part of Earthcare. I am conscious of my limitations as a white settler living in Europe, but also conscious of the responsibility I have of using my education and words to open up ways of listening to Earthothers.

As *Tanganekald, Meintangk, Bunganditj* and *Potaruwutj* legal Scholar Irene Watson states:

> We need to listen to the natural world constantly; now it is changing, howling, raining and drying up. We need to continually monitor dangerous extractive industries which might damage our natural ecosystems. First Nations have never stopped watching and acting; the non-Indigenous world needs to learn how to reciprocate and share the responsibility we have to the natural world. Perhaps it begins with some deep listening to the Indigenous world.
>
> Watson 2018: 138

In the next chapter we move into the thorny question of responsibilities for future generations, asking who and how many can care for Earth, diving into debates about resources, reproduction, care, planetary boundaries and choices around bearing and caring for children.

4

Caring about Having Babies: Reproductive Rights and Population Ethics

The polar icecaps are melting ... is it ok to have a child?
Meehan Crist 2020: 3.

What we explore in this chapter

In a book that discusses feminist conundrums around care, one of the most difficult issues to consider is the set of questions that swirl around having babies. Who makes choices about if, when or how someone bears (or not) children? Some of the questions asked include: Does having a uterus define the identity of a person because of the capacity to bear children? Who has the right to control conception or contraception? Should people have babies given uncertain futures due to climate change?

These are not easy questions to ask – or answer. Most societies see biological reproduction as defining the female biological and social role. Bearing children defines the success of individuals, families and communities. Society and culture are built around it, and as we saw in the earlier chapter on care work, caring for children is at the heart of social reproduction. Having babies is a deeply political question. In the last decades heated global scientific and popular debates around the population, gender and environmental nexus have deeply divided feminists.

In this chapter I explore some of the feminist debates about having babies, starting with 'Birth Stories', my own reflections on having a uterus and making choices about having babies. In Section Two, 'The choice to parent', I look at the conundrums that feminists raise as they share why they care about having babies in the face of climate change. In Section Three, 'Kinning', I look at recent feminism, science and technology studies debates raging around the issue of population and environment and the controversy around the proposal of 'make kin not babies'.

Section One: *Birth stories*

As a feminist it is perplexing to write about choices around having babies. It seems at once an enormously important subject and yet also a trap. I keep wondering whether by focusing on motherhood and babies I play into conservative views about women's place and roles as mothers, confirming the biological determinism of women's maternal role. As Sophie Lewis states, 'what makes a womb-bearing person's life worth living derives directly and solely from the productivity she achieves with that organ, is an idea that dies hard' (Lewis 2017, 193).

It is a question I have puzzled about for decades. My BA Hons thesis was on the 'tyranny of the uterus' looking at hysteria and fashionably ill heroines in nineteenth-century British novels. My PhD was on medical discourses on the female body looking at when gynecology and obstetrics was established in late nineteenth-century Australia. I dug deep into literature and medical texts to understand why and how womanhood was primarily defined by the biological ability to carry a child. In my studies I have continually questioned the politics of motherhood as the defining feature of womanhood, but in my own life it remains a conundrum. As the oldest child of four in a comfortable middle-class white Australian family, I was brought up to think that having children should be a defining part of my life. I never questioned whether I would have children, though I was determined to decide for myself, how and when.

I was lucky. I had my two daughters in a birthing chair, in a Rome clinic, watching the clock, breathing through the pain. Two memorable and momentous times of unforgettable suffering, joy and fulfilment. The care and love for my daughters have shaped my life.

I viscerally found myself reflecting on those personal choices, and the politics of birth and care, when I participated in my younger daughter's art project on the uterus a few years ago. The project was held in an old diamond factory in Amsterdam where she was squatting with friends. I recall arriving at the building, then picking my way through the splintered wood and old furniture she and her friends had dragged in from the street, to arrive at the roof top and a large pink uterus constructed from canvas, ceramics and paint. The project was for her to spend twenty-four hours in the uterus talking with loved ones whom she invited to visit her (in person or by phone). In the darkening sky the uterus was framed in shadows thrown by the nearby church spires and tops of trees. We sat quietly drinking the wine I had brought, as she spoke about her art project. She was full of curiosity about how she was going to be reborn in this event, which she wanted to be spontaneous and natural. I smiled. Those words resonated with my own desire for her and her sister's birth.

I wondered what it meant for me to be natural and spontaneous at this moment, as her mother, listening to my grown daughter's exploration of birth stories. I kept forgetting to inhabit my mother role as we spoke. I was back in my memories, like her, a twenty-something young woman.

At 1.25 am, the time she had been born, she stepped into the uterus. I had agreed to sit alongside her for the night, wrapped in a sleeping bag. I was the first person to accompany her during the twenty-four hours. The mood shifted when she disappeared into the uterus. I spoke more seriously about my pregnancy – how I had almost lost her when I was six weeks pregnant and had stayed in bed for a month until the placenta had reattached. I told her of that time of anxiety and our family's collective work to keep her in my uterus. Her older sister, then three years old, would climb into bed with me so we could eat our meals together. I described how her grandmother sat by my bedside as she sewed an elaborate tapestry of Noah and his animals, now framed on my study wall, which she finished the day my daughter was born. I spoke of how her father drove a car for the last time in his life, to be with me when she was born. She was born very quickly. My cervix had dilated to 8 cm before I felt any pain. She was a strong robust baby. From the minute of her birth, she was her own self; her sweetness hidden in her strength.

As the dampening air pulled around us, we shared our memories and hopes for the future. I relived the care, the pain and love of giving birth.

Eventually I fell asleep by her uterus cocoon, the church clocks of Amsterdam keeping the time for us. I woke at 5 am to gentle, but persistent rain. I staggered awake, woozy from lack of sleep to find something to cover the rain-soaked uterus. In the squat full of junk, I found a rainbow-coloured canvas which I draped over my daughter in what was now a very damp uterus. I ferried towels and extra covers into its aperture. My daughter's face peeking out looked forlorn and tired, but when she was more or less dry, she went back to sleep. At 7 am I heard footsteps on the roof top; her next loved one had arrived. I touched her sleeping shape goodbye before hastening out into the morning air.

I was moved I had been invited to be part of her project. It took me back to her original birth, and I felt again the immensity of having a uterus that carried life. At the same time, it was a project about letting go and seeing her move into her own adult life. The night of talking, watching, being, reliving and sharing shifted what kind of care I could give her. As her adult life evolves, I need to learn to be with her and yet also nourish space and distance to enable us to both to relate and grow as separate beings.

I am aware that this birth story is heteronormative and specific to the privileges and choices I could make, as well as the special bonds I could build with my feminist daughter. I could tell other stories I have heard and seen in my life about harrowing painful births, unwanted pregnancies, miscarriages, abortions, lack of choice, obstetric violence, alienation, bodily harm, mothers and babies that do not survive. I am aware it is not only women who have uteruses, and not all women can carry children. How we make sense of birth experiences depends on 'the contingencies of biology as well as those of time and place, gender, class and race' (Crist 2020: 1). Those experiences are the undercurrent of my own birth stories and shape my sense of gratitude and awe of the birth process and what the female body can do, and how crucial it is to provide support for all bodies to have dignified, healthy pregnancies and safe births.

Section Two: *The choice to parent*

We now move forward from over a quarter of a century ago, when I was making choices about having children, to today's choice to parent, which reflects a decided shift in western popular and academic discourse. The question of whether to have or not have babies given climate crisis is the subject of an increasing number of surveys, high level opinion pieces and novels. While there is still a strong focus on fertility technology and IVF including IVF tourism,[1] progressive papers such as the *Guardian* are highlighting that climate anxiety has extended to people in richer countries deciding, for the good of climate and the future of humanity, *not* to have children. The *Guardian* in May 2024 (Carrington 2024: np) surveyed 843 lead authors of the reports of the Intergovernmental Panel on Climate Change, the data collected since 2018. A fifth of the female climate experts (from Brazil, Chile, Germany, India and Kenya) who responded said they had chosen to have no children or fewer children, due to environmental crises. According to the *Guardian* article they did not wish to add 'to the global human population that is exacting a heavy environmental toll on the planet' (ibid.). Others expressed fears about the climate chaos that their children will inherit. A German professor is quoted as saying that she chose to have one child, but now 'I feel guilty about leaving her in this world without my protection, and guilty about having played a part in the changing climate.' An Indian climate scientist explained she adopted children because 'we are not so special that our genes need to be transmitted: values matter more' (ibid.). A 2020 study of privileged US people (88% of whom were educated white, 70% liberal and 93% graduates) aged 27 to 45 found that most were concerned about the wellbeing of children in a climate-changed world. The authors described how almost 100% were 'concerned about the carbon footprint of procreation' (Schneider-Mayerson and Ling Leong 2020: 1012) and 96.5% of respondents were 'very' or 'extremely concerned' about the wellbeing of their existing, expected or hypothetical children in a climate-changed world (ibid., 1007). The study pointed to 'parental anxiety about how their children will fare in a climate-changed future' with parents regretting having children. They give the example of a 40-year-old teacher and mother in Minnesota who states, 'I regret having my kids because I am terrified that they will be facing the end of the world due to climate change' (ibid., 1015).

Such studies show how middle-class educated people are expressing a general anxiety and fear around having children. The conundrum is extensively discussed by feminist writers. Meehan Crist, in a 2020 article in the *London Review of Books*, puts the question boldly: 'the polar icecaps are melting . . . is it ok to have a child?' (Crist 2020: 3).

As she points out, having children, if you want one, couldn't or didn't have one as a biological parent, is a question all of us ask at some point in our lives. But the shift in our lifetimes is that we now are no longer sure if the (unevenly distributed) conditions for human flourishing will 'reliably exist' (ibid., 2). Her widely read article details the impact of knowing climate risk and ecological disaster have already impacted many people's lives – we have passed tipping points. To have a child is not only about fulfilling intimate desires, but also a 'political act' that evokes 'not only the complex biopolitics of pregnancy and birth but also the intersecting legacies of colonialism, racism and patriarchy' (ibid., 3). The conundrum of care when having a child in the Global North is that it is both a personal and yet a global concern. But as Crist points out, this ignores much of the realities of baby making in the rest of the world and the fact that children born in the Global South already endure the impacts of climate crisis.

While ecological limits are real, she warns that linking ecological disaster with reducing population feeds into population control policies and worse. She points out that the narrative that the individual is personally responsible for the climate crisis has been honed by the fossil fuel industry: 'fossil fuel companies are trying to appear serious about addressing the climate crisis while planning for a future of increased demand' (Crist 2020: 8). For Crist, 'it is dangerous to assume we know what the limits are and to start curbing births accordingly' (ibid., 11). She suggests that the choice we need to make is not whether to eat meat or how many children to have, but how to make profound structural changes 'without which no personal choices will matter' (ibid.). She suggests that humanity has not yet tried to exist sustainably on this planet. We therefore need to hold onto the hopeful possibility that 'human flourishing could happen in unprecedented and as yet unimaginable circumstances' (ibid., 14). In the article Crist shares her son's birth story, while stating you do not have to give birth to believe in the possibility of a human future which 'will always be more terrible and wonderful than any of us can possibly imagine' (ibid., 16).

In a personal reflection on the choice to have children, Elizabeth Rush tells the story of her trip to Thwaites Glacier in the Antarctica on a scientific mission aboard the research vessel R/V Nathaniel B. Palmer in January 2019. The book opens with the author's mother describing Rush's birth, and throughout the book we hear stories from the other fifty-six people on the boat about their birth, or their children's birth or their concerns around whether to have children given climate change. For example, one scientist states: 'My work on Thwaites feeds into a general unease that I carry around about the future. There's this really basic question: Is it a sensible choice to have kids at this point? I'm afraid of messed-up politics ...' (Rush 2023: 83).

These stories run alongside Rush's own guilty thoughts about her deep desire to have a child: 'What if I also give up what I have been told is one of the most meaningful human experiences? Might that sacrifice be big enough to make things better?' (ibid., 104). Alongside the different birth stories is the communal concern about the impact of climate change on the glaciers the scientists are responsible for observing. The two narratives of birth stories merge as the glaciers are seen as calving icebergs in an extraordinary landscape. As Rush describes it: 'the ocean coils up into a round wave, making the seam where the ice sheet meets the bay looking as though it is bending into a massive blue arch' (ibid., 292). The beauty of the icebergs forming contrasts starkly with their scientific measurements, which reveal how much the impact of human activities is inexorably speeding up the melting of the glacier.

The book captures anxiety about the climate crisis and what Rush describes as the '[r]age at what it denies parents who need the transformation of our energy systems now, so their children might face fewer risks in a climate-changed world. Rage that my own desire to have children has always, for as long as I can remember, filled me simultaneously with joy and fear and guilt. Rage at the time I lost, feeling ashamed for wanting to become a mother' (ibid., 71). After the trip Rush does have a son, during the Covid-19 lockdown in the US, which though all went well, reads as a harrowing birth experience.

Her book weaves together the difficult labour of living in and imagining a changed world; one which her son will inherit. The book resonated with my on-going discussions with my daughters, who want children but are not sure of the world they would bring them into. They too express rage at the people of my generation who so carelessly destroyed the planet with their thoughtless desires and avid consumption.

These writings are framed within an educated middle class (mostly white) western sense of individual possibilities and ideas of choice. The conundrum is whether we can justify our desire to have children at the cost of the health of the planet. Moving to where communities depend on children for their livelihoods, the conundrum changes to who can afford not to have children? Having children gives meaning to a life everywhere, but in poorer communities, particularly in rural areas, children are integral to survival, livelihoods, status, culture and the future. But here the choices to parent are couched in the literature not as individual choices, but rather framed in population numbers codified in technological, economic and ecological terms related to economic policy (Silliman and King 1999; Sasser 2018; Wilson 2019).

Jade Sasser (2024) calls attention to the arguments of reproductive justice and the importance of listening to marginalised peoples' experiences of populationism, which is determining their parenting choices. The reproductive justice framing emerges from the struggles of women of colour in the US and feminists from the Global South against racialised experiences of forcible sterilisation and promotion of unsafe contraceptives (Silliman and King 1999; Wilson 2017; Sasser 2018).[2] It is explicitly against population interventions such as coerced sterlisation, contraceptive testing and reduced access to reproductive health for racialised communities, and questions 'ideologies that attribute social and ecological ills to human numbers' (Sasser 2024: 2). These are, Sasser argues, based on racist assumptions that 'women of colour have too many children, are irresponsible parents, or have too few resources to raise their children well' (ibid.). They reject 'framings that position population size and growth as a driver of social, political, economic, and environmental problems' (ibid.). Reproductive justice advocates are worried that climate change has reanimated Malthusian concerns that link population trends and environmental problems in narratives about resource conservation, sustainability and agricultural productivity (Sasser 2018: 2024). Population growth in the Global South is linked to climate change, continuing to blame the poor rather than calling attention to systemic inequalities of neoliberal capitalism and devoid of any recognition of wider local, national and global structures of power (Wilson 2017). The conundrum is that framing this as reproductive choice or raising concerns about the environmental responsibilities to have or not have children obscures structural inequalities of power and resources.

Discourses that argue for a reduction of numbers due to limited planetary resources are haunted by the Malthusian spectre of scarcity (Mehta 2010: 11). Calling attention to the problem of scarce resources due to population numbers ignores the geo-political, economic and social relations which determine the access to resources. As Lyla Mehta (2010) points out, 'the conception of scarcity has been politicized, naturalized, and universalized in academic and policy debates' (ibid., 3) so that we see planetary limits as an overall concern about scarcity rather than understanding who creates scarcity and who benefits from it. Climate change in these debates is about scarcity of fuel, water and energy in a totalising discourse where local knowledges and experiences are ignored along with understandings of how power is distributed. Should limits be set for all, no matter what resources you consume? Or should the question be 'who is consuming what' and therefore 'for whom should there be limits?' And the vital question is 'who sets these limits and thresholds?' (ibid., 5). In poor rural contexts in the Global South where people struggle to survive, it is not possible to understand choices in terms of dominant western notions of family, children and individualised self-fulfilment. Having children is engrained into family and community social and economic survival. The concerns here should not be about reducing numbers but about access to resources (material, economic, legal and health) and questions about fairer distribution of resources in increasingly extractive and ecologically damaged environments. Not to mention the questions to be asked about the cultural, economic and social discrimination against women who do not have children.

Section Three: *Kinning*

These concerns around scarcity and population belong to a long legacy of debates about the impact of human population size on the environment. From eugenics to theories of the population bomb, population programme policies in the nineteenth and twentieth centuries have had a profound impact on marginalised people in the Global South, with population control measures being applied through questionable incentives and at times by force. Infamous examples of population control programmes are Indira Gandhi's 1970s programmes of forced vasectomy in regional India and the scandal around injectable contraceptives, such as depo-provera, taken off the shelf in richer countries and being used in family planning programmes in the Pacific and parts of Africa.[3]

Betsy Hartmann's (1995) *Reproductive Rights and Wrongs: The Global Politics of Population Control* set out the widely accepted transnational feminist position that counters Malthusian population policy practices. The international UN Conference on Population and Development held in Cairo in 1994 established women's choice as central to sexual and reproductive health and rights (Harcourt 2009). The feminist position on reproductive justice, which emerged from debates before and after the Cairo conference, closely scrutinised the use of population numbers in environmental policy. The argument was that the issue was not about how many the planet can hold but about halting the damage of a greedy few. Instead of governments seeking to control the numbers of children of families in the Global South, governments should stop people in the Global North using up the resources. Feminists point to the inherent sexism, racism and classism of population policy. Environmental and intergenerational justice should be about 'social-environmental process required to maintain everyday life and to sustain human cultures and communities on a daily basis and intergenerationally' (Di Chiro 2008: 281), not about telling women how many children they should have. Bhatia et al. (2020) label the pernicious birth control policies as populationism or ways of 'understanding and addressing social and environmental problems' in a form of Malthusianism that 'produce, reinforce, and naturalize inequalities along lines of race, class, gender and place ... in strategies across the political right and left' (Bhatia et al. 2020: 336).

Such conversations around population are fraught with concerns about human rights, racism, colonialism and ideological differences, 'entangled with contested definitions of sexuality, gender roles and identities, family norms and embodiment, as well as with ideological disputes over the role of the state and its powers' (Coole 2018: 4). Feminists have continued to be concerned that choices for women are undermined by racialised assumptions that black and brown bodies need to be constrained from having too many children for the sake of the environment, even if the environmental impact of 'human numbers are nearly impossible to tease out because they are not, and never have been, simply biological – they are the result of biological, and political, and economic, and technological, and cultural processes and practices' (Sasser 2018: 150). As Sasser states, the assumption that 'population growth is a threat to nature and the environment does not in fact reflect an essential, immutable biological reality. Instead, it reflects long-standing debates among scientists, activists, academics, and policymakers working to define problems and how to solve them' (Sasser 2010: 50).

There have been several heated debates in feminism, science and technology studies when Donna Haraway made a controversial push for 'making kin not babies' if we are to support life on Earth and find new liveable forms of sustainable justice. Many feminists were shocked at Haraway's foray into the debate. They question 'how her call for 'multispecies ecojustice' is compatible with a vision for reproductive justice when her provocative slogan 'Make Kin Not Babies!' accompanies a vision of a desired future in which 'human people of this planet can again be numbered two or three billion' (Bhatia et al. 2020: 336). Haraway's idea that growing human numbers are linked to environmental degradation was seen as 'populationist' betraying 'feminist, cultural, and science studies' (Subramaniam 2018). Feminists were concerned that Haraway's *Making Kin Not Babies* (2014 and 2016) and *Making Kin Not Population* (2013), appearing twenty years after Cairo, could feed into growing conservative arguments that we are too many for the planet as governments try to grapple with climate change, environmental degradation, international migration and increasing poverty. Haraway boldly stated: we need to 'find ways to celebrate low birth rates and personal, intimate decisions to make flourishing and generous lives (including innovating enduring kin – kinnovating) without making more babies urgently and especially, but not only, in wealthy high-consumption and misery-exporting regions, nations, communities, families, and social classes' (Haraway 2016: 164).

Haraway decentres the human in her multispecies politics of reproductive justice when she argues that humans do not need to seek fulfilment by having human children. If reproductive justice is about collective thriving – including environmental justice, food justice, climate justice, antiracist social justice – it requires humans to reduce their numbers to end the violent ways humans relate to the planet. Making kin (not babies) is about being caring and responsible for all living beings. Sustaining life should not be about genes, inheritance and family but about creating relations of care, mutual interdependence and solidarity with people and other species. Such a forging of connections, Haraway argues, is more ethically important than making (fostering, surrogating) babies. Haraway troubles the growth of the human population because it is exacerbating the environmental crisis. She presents her arguments as ethical and political responses, told through 'narrative speculative fabulation' which imagine future technologies that merge human and more-than-human forms (Haraway 2016: 55).

Her essays ask feminists to value nonhuman kin as part of the feminist project to unpack corporate power, technoscience and biopolitics. Her imaginative speculative fiction envisages a feminist forging of multi-species ecojustice that breaks through the gendered and racialised nature of biology, culture and technology.

Feminists like Hartmann, Sasser and Ojeda respond with deep concern that such speculative fiction by a prominent feminist could play into a renewed justification for the control of racialised bodies in environment policy (Hartmann 1998; Ojeda et al. 2019; Sasser 2014) as well as denying women's needs and desires to have children, particularly in the Global South. Their concern is that the 'population problem' in the context of climate change has resulted in the 'gendering of environmental culprits' and a failure of 'reproductive justice' as women bodies, particularly impoverished and racialised women's bodies, 'have been targeted by population control measures' (Ojeda et al. 2019: 327). They provide a rationale for intervening in ways that conceal and reinforce systems of power and inequality (Bhatia et al.

2020: 336). Sasser labels this 'feminist populationism' (2024: 6) and questions Haraway's call for multispecies ecojustice, which reduced biological reproduction in unexplained ways which Sasser argues evades the need to redress social inequality for marginalised groups, even if claiming an opposition to coercion.

I recently set out my own response to feminist populationism in a conversation with one of my PhD students (Fenner and Harcourt 2023). We argue that it is not about a simple yes or no to having babies, but about the ethics required to inform such a decision. It is one thing to decide not to have children because I can kin with neighbouring people, animals, trees or landscapes. It is another to be coerced into not having children for the good of the planet. The focus on how many people the planet can carry directs attention away from the need for the redistribution of resources, including drastic changes in rich people's lifestyles and who has the power to decide for whom. More global pandemics and unbearable living conditions due to climate change could well lead to inequitable policies if we do not acknowledge the racial, colonial and patriarchal discourses underlying state biopolitics. It is important to embed population studies in the broader political and social conundrums. Too often, demographers do not perceive their work as political but rather as empirical truths about changing population trends and patterns. Such assumptions can lead to policies which propose that the reduction in population numbers is the way to conserve the environment (Harcourt 2020). For me the issue is not about 'how many people' but about distribution and justice. Whether the planet's carrying capacity is 3 or 11 or 20 billion people is not the point – far more powerful and important are the multiple and complex interrelationships that raw numbers can obfuscate. Progressive politics should be about distribution of resources, changes in rich people's lifestyles and openness to all women's reproductive choices, full stop, not a set of 'population' policies that aim to reduce numbers because too many (poor) people cause too much environmental damage. Diversity and context matter. We need to be aware of who can access what resources and who is deciding what constitutes too many. I remain worried about how this is all playing out, particularly given the crazy and unpredictable global geo-politics of Trump 2. I fear that the likelihood of regular global pandemics and heat waves, fires and floods due to climate change will produce an inequitable set of policies if we do not point to racial, colonial and patriarchal discourses underlying current policies and seek very different behaviour (not just good policy).

I remain uncertain about what is the answer and whether it is possible to rethink kinning in a world dominated by numbers that hide the oppression of poor communities, violence towards women's bodies and the uncertain futures we all face. It is an emotive issue that requires discussion but one that is currently ridden with anxieties. Haraway herself appeals to strong emotions when she makes her proposal for kin not babies:

> This is a brazenly personal paper and a plea for other-than-biogenetic kindred. I begin with a painful mass in my gut, pressing up against my diaphragm until it ruptures. The pain is much like the bodily feeling of grief when my mother died, when my first husband died, when my father died, when the dog of my heart died – the feeling of grief, exploding from the inside out, evisceration, terror. (. . .) But the pain I feel in my belly has to do with something else (. . .) the surplus killings of ongoingness, the wanton surplus extinction of kinds, of whole patterns of living and dying on earth, of genocides across human and other than human groups.
>
> Haraway, 2018: 69

The passion she feels is palpable. I share that sense of despair that despite so much struggle there is still a lack of contraceptive choice, sexual violence towards women and peoples who do not conform to heterosexual norms, wrapped up in debates around autonomy and sexual health and reproductive rights. I also feel an overwhelming sense of loss of biodiversity. I cannot believe that so many tipping points are here, now. But I deeply regret that young people question if they can have children due to economic uncertainty and climate change. When I decided to have children, it was about how to make an aware set of feminist biological, technological and economic choices. Such 'choices' for my daughters are now entangled in a larger collective sense of social and environmental responsibilities.

These include a growing collective sense of grief as climate crisis is impacting the emotional and mental health of communities worldwide with anxiety, depression, loss, sadness and guilt (Ojala et al. 2021; Howard 2022). Environmental melancholia and environmental grief lead to people feeling overwhelmed and anxious about having children with 'reproductive anxieties' on emotional, moral and ethical levels (Sasser 2024: 9).

Climate activist groups bring these climate-reproductive questions to the public arena as an issue of intergenerational justice. In the Global North there is an emerging parent-led climate justice movement that aims to address intergenerational climate responsibilities. These communities act both from a sense of fear as well as from hope and solidarity in their collective actions. Lisa Howard describes how in these communities 'interactions with fellow activists were a crucial source of communal, supportive feelings to counter uncomfortable emotions of fear and frustration' (Howard 2022: 4). Such ecoparent groups overlap with other environmental movements such as Transition Towns, Greenpeace, Extinction Rebellion and Women's Environmental Network (ibid., 3). As such they are not just acting as individual parents, but as politicised citizens aware of the structural impediments to action and how race and class as well as gender and age interact in affective responses to climate injustice in activist spaces. Climate anxiety has been seen as an overwhelmingly white phenomena, but as climate crisis continues the storms, floods, droughts, fires and heat events globally, the emotional responses by communities along the lines of race, class, gender and geography will intensify (Ray 2021).

Conundrums of having babies

Haraway's question about 'how to celebrate human maturity for women and men in building selves and communities without making babies?' (Haraway 2018: 97) remains for me a conundrum. The communities I have been part of, whether activist, academic or friendship-based (and sometimes all three), have been key to my adult maturity, but I still see having children as profoundly defining my life. I also look to the environments around me, whether they are the oceans in Australia or the lakes in Italy or the woods in the Netherlands or even the plants and flowers on my terrace. While I can tentatively call this kinning, as their presence offers a tiny way to help me face the overwhelming emotions of our dark times, I realise Haraway's call is not one I am truly answering.

Part of the reason for finding kinning a difficult conversation is that while a plea for other-than-biogenetic kindred is important, the appeal to multispecies justice appears not to acknowledge the current struggles of reproductive justice for marginalised and racialised people. Feminists need to be aware of the power and privilege that 'shapes national and transnational commodified markets in bodies, babies, and reproductive labor' (Jolly 2016: 73). We need to tread carefully.

In the next chapter we turn to the question of interspecies care.

5

Interspecies Care: Learning with the More-than-Human

How can we listen across species, across extinction, across harm?
Alexis Pauline Gumbs 2020: 14.

What we explore in this chapter

Chapter 4 concluded with the conundrum of whether Donna Haraway's proposal to make kin not babies was a troubling form of populationism or a radical form of multispecies justice. We pick up the theme of multispecies justice in this chapter as we delve further into interspecies care and human responsibilities for more-than-human relations. In the first section I share companion stories about the menagerie I enjoyed in my childhood. Section Two discusses interspecies justice in feminist writings in the humanities and social sciences, looking into why we need to care about human entanglements with the more-than-human beings. The third section reflects on caring responses to toxic environments in the writings and approaches of ecofeminism, black feminist ecology and queer ecology, learning about more-than-human relations in complex histories of racism, power differences, subversion and loss.

Section One: *Companion stories*

I grew up in the late 1960s and 1970s in a rambling urban household of four children, two parents and a host of more-than-human others.

We had Rocky the budgerigar, who lived in the kitchen and would energetically mimic our noisy family discussions. There were two white female rabbits in the back garden that made love in the moonlight. My father tended an aviary full of brightly coloured love birds, finches, mulga parrots and rosellas that fluttered among the rough wood shelving with tiny brown quails running along the grassy edges. We had green and yellow canaries that sung in a cage in the shade of the verandah. Families of caged white mice and brown and black hamsters did their turn on wheels in the shed. Cats came and went, with my favourite, a black tortoiseshell, Inky, surviving to die peacefully at 18 years old in the shade of a large gum tree in our front garden. A pink and grey galah, caught by my father the day one of my brothers was born, would call out 'pretty cocky want a cracker' when you passed by his cage. And we had one short-lived rescue dog, Ben, a basenji that tried to outrace cars and met a fatal end.

We loved our co-existence with these creatures. My father had a passion for birds and would get up early morning in his pyjamas to feed them seeds and green leafy vegetables. We trailed behind him, careful not to disturb any nesting females. We were not flaunting any laws then, but now native species birds are not allowed to be kept privately, and modern sensibilities question keeping birds and animals in cages for human enjoyment. As much as we could we took care of our pets, but I have horrid memories of not only our dog being run over, and cats disappearing, but also of baby mice dying in the heat, hamsters frozen dead on the wheel, and our galah, with one last squawk, dying as he was removed from the cage as he was given to a friend who was to look after him when we were going overseas.

This troubling if homely story of living with the more-than-human beings belongs to a particular time and place and shows the conundrum of how difficult and ethically suspect it is to forge relations of human companionship with other species in modern western life. As an adult I have limited my companion species relations. I write this with Pancho, a loveable fluffy black dog asleep under my desk. I have learnt to see him not so much as our family dog, but as a person in his own right who requires care. We have reciprocal needs, Pancho and me. He provides me respite from my tendency to overwork, I provide him shelter and food. Together we enjoy long walks in the woods and on the beach and we keep each other company in the evenings. His care is shared with my daughter, who provides him with a more exciting life of travel with her adventurous friends. Pancho is a chill and happy little dog, but still I am uncomfortably aware how he was bred and is trained to meet human needs.

The thrill of being touched by wild, untamed creatures gives quite a different feeling. In the summer of 2024, I was visiting a beautiful shrine in Kyoto, Japan, where spiritual meaning is imbued in the delicate and ornate buildings and stunning gardens that are arranged so that each view takes your breath away. I was walking down one of the ambling paths leading away from the shrine when a butterfly alighted on my arm and travelled with me as I made my way down, fanning itself, until I placed it, some minutes later, on a bush of flowers. I felt a connection with the butterfly and was grateful for its friendly gesture that resonated with the spiritual atmosphere created by the aesthetic of the shrine and gardens. While I feel coy in sharing this story, it is an attempt to pay attention to relations with more-than-human beings and to consider how animals, plants, soil, mountains and water play vital roles in our lives that cannot be captured by scientific measurements alone.

My small stories skim lightly towards what Anna Tsing calls 'arts of noticing' that aim to understand how 'the lives of beings matter to each other in distinct and complicated ways, when they become entangled in shared cosmopolitical worlds' (Chao et al. 2022: 247).

Section Two: *Interspecies entanglements*

In recent years there has been a proliferation of research in the arts, humanities and social sciences looking at questions of more-than-human agency and at the ways animals and plants and other beings constitute our complex, multispecies worlds. Feminist ethics on care have produced new methodologies for 'immersive' knowledge (Tsing 2011: 9) with more-than-humans, which have inspired research on how to learn with beings in 'other worlds' (van Doreen 2018: 60). These methods of knowing and learning include art practices, journalling life with other species, and experiments in innovative forms of ethical research with more-than-human others. In this section we reflect on how feminist writing about ethics of care invites us to think differently about interspecies care; subverting dominant hierarchies which place humans above other species. We consider the conundrum of how we care for other-than-human-beings (plants, animals, earth elements) as *affect*, looking at how 'sensual qualities of being and the capacity to experience and understand the world in profoundly relational and productive ways' (Liljeström 2015: 16) impact and shape our ways of being.

Three outstanding feminist scholars, Anna Tsing, Catriona Sandilands and Maria Puig de la Bellacasa, provide ways to navigate the ethics of caring for more-than-human others in their work on care, ethics and politics in relation to plants and soil. Their investigations into interspecies entanglements look at humans as one among other forms of life caught up in diverse relationships of knowing and living together. Their writing pushes us beyond anthropocentricism. They point to the lively ways the boundaries between humans and other life forms are porous and intertwined.

Feminist anthropologist Anna Tsing, in her multispecies ethnography on mushrooms, speaks of her and other peoples' research that engages in 'passionate immersion in the lives of the nonhuman subjects being studied' (Tsing 2010: 201). She combines the 'learnedness in natural science' with humanities and the arts to encourage 'public imagination to make new ways of relating to nature possible' (ibid.). Her profoundly influential book *The mushroom at the end of the world* (2015) critiques the global economy through her immersive study of the matsutake mushroom. She connects global economic activity to human cultural dimensions of mushroom foraging, exporting and consumption and the entanglement of fungi, pine trees and nematodes with the lives of the people in northern Finland, China's Yunnan Province, Oregon, US and Japan. Her journey follows the Matsutake mushroom through the entangled relations of pines, forest, landscape, humans, foraging, gift cultures, trading paths and economic practices.

From Tsing's story of the matsutake we learn of ways to understand the complexity of human relations with more-than-human species in our precarious and uncertain times. Guided by her sense of hope about how a mushroom can emerge from degraded landscapes, Tsing acknowledges that while we are facing 'trouble without end', we can survive if we exercise curiosity and hope (Tsing 2015: 2). Tsing's research on the matsutake shows 'possibilities of coexistence with environmental disturbance' (ibid., 4).

The conundrum of how to face crisis with hope is a strong theme in feminist writings on interspecies care. Queer ecologist Catriona Sandilands brings together ecology, gender and sexuality in her writings on biopolitics.[1] We need to see 'beauty in the wounds of the world' and take 'responsibility to care for the world as it is' (Mortimer-Sandilands 2005: 24, quoted in Di Chiro 2010: 200). Sandilands coined the term 'queer ecologies' to describe the connections among sexuality, nature and power in ecological biopolitical relations that govern both humans and plants, and other more-than-human forms of life.

Sandilands studies plants as active agents in our life-worlds. In a 2019 interview she describes her research/relations/connections with

Douglas-firs in the British Columbia Southern Gulf Islands, where she lives half the year (Cielemęcka and Åsberg 2019). She studies trees as complex interspecies beings – through their communication networks and in their economic and political roles as industrial tree species since the colonisation of British Columbia. She describes how her life with Douglas-Firs is not only about research but also about her sensuous and political entangled relations with the species that provide shelter and aesthetic experiences – her log cabin is built from the Firs and looks out into forests of the tall green trees.

Sandilands positions herself as a caretaker on the stolen land of the Gulf Islands, which is 'a shadow of its former, botanically-rich self by a combination of dispossession, development, and deer' (Sandilands 2021: 777). Part of her place-based research is to restore plant communities for future human caretakers. She is conscious of her temporal space – readying for climate change – anticipating that plants, animals and humans will need to be able to withstand temperature extremes and lack of water. She attributes agency to plants as 'world makers ... forces of life ... world defenders ... especially on this warming planet ... they hold and keep other elements in balance' (ibid., 778).

In explaining why relations with plants matter to humans, Sandilands brings a sharp awareness of the problem of 'plant blindness' (Wandersee and Schussler 1999) in western, urbanised settings. The systemic insensitivity to plants is partly because plants move in different scales and temporalities from human beings, and also because many plants we eat come packaged in supermarkets rather than growing in nearby trees or soil. For most urban dwellers plants are a green backdrop to our busy lives. She calls on us to redress that alienation and pay attention to plants by tending specific plant relationships. Following queer black feminist Alexis Pauline Gumbs, Sandilands suggests we *identify* with plants and 'practice humanity with some of that world-making plantiness folded inside', which might help us as humans to be not so 'tangled in [the] separation and domination that it is consistently making our lives incompatible with the planet' (Gumbs 2020: 9). Sandilands shares her deeply felt intergenerational and interspecies connection with plants in a heart-rendering story of her mother's love of plants even in the throes of dementia, and how Sandilands continues to care for her mother's beloved jade plants and aloes 'because it matters to be able to continue the care' (Sandilands 2021: 779).

Maria Puig de la Bellacasa, in her iconic *Matters of care* (2017), offers one of the most expansive feminist texts on care for thinking and living in more-than-human worlds.[2] She sees human and nonhuman relations of care as deeply entangled with ethical and affective implications for our future lives. Her work investigates the 'meanings of care for knowing and thinking with more than human worlds in technoscience and naturecultures' (Puig de la Bellacasa 2017: 3). It feels presumptuous to pull out just a few insights from such a beautifully argued book, but in terms of interspecies relations her work on soil (which she is continuing to research) is particularly powerful. In the last chapter of the book she analyses ecological practices that are 'rematering soil from inert, usable substance and resource into a living world of which humans are also part' (ibid., 4). She presents the novel idea that if we are to survive climate catastrophe, we need to disrupt productivist future-oriented technoscience by making time to take care of our ecological relations with soil.

Puig de la Bellacasa's reflections on soil start from the scientific and policy discourses on the damage to soil due to industrialised and unsustainable forms of agriculture, and intensifying food production (ibid., 169). Scientific reports address the growing environmental disasters such as desertification, food insecurity and climate change, underlining that soil requires global care. Puig de la Bellacasa warns that such global care should not be driven by the dominant productivist vision that treats soil only as a vehicle for commodifiable produce, where worn-out soils must be 'put back to work' through soil engineering technologies to increase soil's efficiency (ibid., 186). She points to how such a focus is at the expense of all other species relations. Soil ecology has countered this approach since the 1990s, analysing soil as a living multispecies world rather than a mere receptacle for crops. Soil ecology presents human-soil relations in a foodweb model which analyses soil as a multispecies community of organisms of biota such as algae, bacteria, fungi, protozoa, nematodes, arthropods, earthworms and larger animals such as rabbits and plants. Puig de la Bellacasa argues that seeing 'soils as a living multispecies world involve[s] changes in the ways humans maintain, care, and foster this liveliness' (ibid., 191).[3] In this vision, human-soil relations of care are where humans are 'members' of the soil community rather than 'consumers of its produce or beneficiaries of its services' (ibid., 192).

The foodweb model based on caring relations with soil recognises vital relations of interdependency between humans and soil. Humans need to engage in the work of care for creating liveable and lively worlds that recognise their entanglement with organisms in soil based on 'material, ethical, and affective ecologies' (Puig de la Bellacasa 2017: 203): 'all of us who benefit from the life in the soil, [need to] become obliged to worms and other Earth creatures for their work' (ibid., 220). By acknowledging the need for relations of care in more-than-human living ecologies in 'situated ecological terrains' of different soils (ibid., 220), care becomes a vital practice for interspecies justice. Relations with soils are part of the 'concrete work of maintenance, with ethical and affective implications' in our interdependent worlds (ibid., 3). The dependency of the (human) carer on soil is 'not so much from soil's produce or 'service' but from an inherent relationality' (ibid., 192). Her analysis rematters soil from inert, usable resource into a living interspecies world of which humans are also part. Her work has inspired studies that have looked at how relational ethics is shaping soils as humans learn to attend and be responsible for the more-than-human other, in care networks of interrelations, connections and dependencies (Krzywoszynska 2019: 664).

These are urgent matters of care when you consider that The Lancet Commission on pollution and health in 2018 found that 61 million people in the 49 countries surveyed are exposed to heavy metals and toxic chemicals at contaminated sites, yet soil pollution is rarely recognised as a pressing environmental concern (Ureta et al. 2022: 1). Research of vulnerable communities exposed to soil pollution has used citizen science as a methodology to support communities living with the many forms of soil pollution caused by the industrial production and mineral extraction. The project *Nuestros Suelos* (Our Soil) in Chile is an example of citizen-led research that is reimagining ways for technoscience to engage with the public and make visible soil pollution.[4]

There is an increasing number of studies on interspecies care engaging with the work of Haraway, Tsing, Sandilands and Puig de la Bellacasa.[5] I found it fascinating that recent debates around the nature and practice of care involving more-than-human relations have extended to the complexities of care with 'awkward creatures', such as insects that bite and sting yet also intrigue (Bear 2021). Research on shifting notions of 'care' and responsibility in insect farming asks how insects can be recognised as active in their caregiving processes, and what this might mean for humanity's ethical relations with insects as they are now being seen as harvestable food (Yee and Sharp 2023). The interdependence of humans on insects such as bees, ants and grasshoppers is shifting as they are marketed as alternative human and animal food sources that can reduce socio-environmental degradation as well as provide gastronomical innovation. The writers raise the condundrum on how to extend an ethics of care to insects. How is it possible for insect farmers and insects to reciprocate care, to acknowledge insects as having agents? Can caring for insects be about caring with? As with livestock farming (Krzywoszynska 2019), there are limitations to how much we can care for more-than-human others and how agencies operate in multispecies networks of care (Yee and Sharp 2023: 93). Bear underlines the limitation of care when attending and being responsible to the more-than-human in insect farming (Bear 2021: 1014). Understanding multispecies companionship with 'awkward' creatures such as insects opens questions about the relationship between 'care' and 'ethical regard' for these forms of human life and reminds us that care cannot be reduced to 'a universal set of principles' (Krzywoszynska 2019: 662). Caring involves 'creating the space to affect and be affected', which, in turn, enables animals to '"speak back" in ways that reshape their environment' (Bear 2021: 1016).

These studies show that care is also about practical work for specific lives/things in specific places, at specific times. While interspecies justice and the foodweb model bring all cares together, there are still different forms of care required. As Mol et al. (2010) stresses, care is always multiple, and often in tension. Wellbeing for one species inevitably encroaches on the wellbeing of another entity. While Puig de la Bellacasa invites us to acknowledge human rootedness in soils as a way to form a symbiotic relationship with soil, Krzywoszynska (2019) asks how can human practices adapt to whatever may count as needs of soils? As in livestock farming, there is an inevitable tension between 'caring, controlling and killing' (ibid., 662).

Another intriguing collection of essays on *Care and belonging in a relational world* (2017)[6] examines how human lives are processes inherently intertwined in multispecies interactions and multispecies communities. The essays look at diverse practices of care as 'a practice of responsiveness and attentiveness that is always entangled in global economic force fields determining who receives care and at what price' (van Dooren et al. 2017: 7). The storying with more-than-human others, from elephants and seahorses to viruses and crows, explores interspecies care as 'an effort to craft better worlds with others' (ibid., 9).

Thom van Dooren's stories on responsible cohabitation with crows (van Dooren 2017: 60) follow Tsing's immersive practices that grapple with the complexity of the lived world, including death and extinction (van Dooren et al. 2017: 9).[7] His work on other-than-human relations with crows is a practice in multispecies ethics, looking with empathy at forty crows marked for killing as environmental pests in the Hoek van Holland, a small town directly opposite the giant Port of Rotterdam, the largest and busiest port in Europe. The lives of the crows have been entangled for generations with the Port, as progeny of crow stowaways. Van Dooren points to the conundrum that these forty crows are depicted by the Government as a major environmental problem, yet they are positioned next to the Port of Rotterdam with its massive destructive environmental impact. The Port of Rotterdam is a huge petrochemical industrial complex, with vast amounts of polluting cargo transhipment and a transit point for international freights. How can this in-your-face evidence of the catastrophe of the Anthropocene be compared to the environmental impact of forty crows? In his study of crows, Van Dooren unpacks the sustainable development discourse, pointing to how policies of death and extinction are embedded in environmental policy around conservation and development.

Sophie Chao also tackles difficult interspecies stories, looking at the affect of the palm oil. *The shadow of the palms: More-than-human becomings in West Papua* (2022) is based on Chao's years of immersion in the West Papua. Her book tells of grief and loss caused by palm oil in plantations shaped by oppressive colonialism and aggressive State-led agribusiness.

On one level Chao's narrative is about how the cash-crop of oil palm has violently transformed the environment, livelihoods and life-worlds of the Indigenous Marind people in West Papua. On another level it is about interspecies relations among Indigenous sago palm, the introduced oil palms and the Marind people. Chao shows how the

Marind are engaged in a reciprocal caring relationship with the Indigenous Sago palm in a fluid process of 'perceptual transspecies becoming' (Chao 2022: 130) and 'gastro-cultural connections' (ibid., 141). The oil palm disrupts these reciprocal relations, causing damage to the land and waterscapes of the region due to drought, herbicide and pesticide, land clearing and military presence. Chao shows both how palm plantations violently change the landscape and how the Marind community are in relation with the oil palm. They understand the palm as domineering and overwhelming yet living a bleak existence divorced from relations with other species. The Marind see the oil palm as a victim of its usefulness to global neoliberal capitalism. Chao tells her story as part of the end times, but unlike Tsing she is less about hope and more about plantation 'violence' as a multispecies act. At the same time, Chao shows her care, grief and loss and sense of responsibility to the Marind and their doomed landscape. In other writing she does retain hope: '[a]t the frayed edges, perimeters, and in the spaces-between human justices, we just might recognize previously unheard voices of myriad insects, plants, waterways, forests, spores, and other outlaws, singing their own corridos – old songs of love and loss, daring escapes and even little justices: recalled, remembered, lived in and longed for' (Chao et al. 2022: 237).

These writers open possibilities for us to be curious about different forms of interspecies entanglements as we pay attention to how plants, animals, microbes and fungi are intertwined with human social worlds. They offer innovative, sympathetic and passionate imaginings about interspecies care. They present it as vital to humans, who are as ecologically vulnerable as other species and ecosystems. They ask us to consider 'how thinking with and practising care and interspecies kinship might contribute to human and nonhuman cohabiting in livelier multispecies worlds' (Desai and Smith 2018: 42).

Such more-than-human biographical and political lives help us to understand how both human and more-than-human lives are increasingly in danger, but they also offer possibilities for finding ways to live in troubled times, listening and learning from more-than-humans in the spaces-between.

Section Three: *Embodied toxicity*

Pushing deeper into interspecies care we turn in this section to the writings of queer and disability justice theorists and activists, radical ecofeminists and black ecologists, and feminist artists. Their approaches to interspecies care help us to understand and act on our shared 'embodied ecologies' (Di Chiro 2010: 216). The concept 'embodied ecologies' refers to how human bodies are intimately entangled with other bodies and care for those other bodies is a necessary act of survival in a world of waste and toxicants that endure in bodies, even after death. Their writing, visual and performance art and political demands push us to understand interspecies care in relation to toxicity and its impact on diverse bodies.

Mel Y. Chen's work (2012, 2023) opens the possibility of care across the realm of animacy, as toxicity becomes absorbed in human and other bodies due to industrialisation and environmental destruction. She explores how human bodies are intimately connected to other bodies, both animate and inanimate, through polluted air, contaminated water and poisoned food. She argues that all these connections express different gender, sexual, racial and class components because 'toxins participate vividly in the racial mattering of locations, human and nonhuman bodies, living and inert entities' (Chen 2012: 21).

In her book *Animacies* (2012), she reflects on her experience of illness due to mercury poisoning, positioning her body as a site of intimate encounters with environmental contaminants. She writes how living with illness made her pause in order to accept how the slow poisoning of mercury was intimately part of life. She details how her experience of suffering changed her relations to her body and to others. She describes how she became acutely aware of a slowing down of time and a sense of porosity around life and death (ibid., 34). As a queer theorist she analyses how the sense of a 'normal' world order is 'lost when, for instance, things that can harm you permanently are not even visible to the naked eye' (ibid., 203). She invites us to consider how toxins are animating cultural life as she explores human anxieties around life and death in growing environmental devastation. Her point is that these toxic realities require us to practice 'an ethics of care and sensitivity that extends far from humans' own borders' (ibid., 237) as we live with the affects of mercury and other toxins.

In *Intoxicated* (2023) Chen continues these conversations as she explores the on-going relationship between race, sexuality and disability as part of imperialism. In her discussion of toxicity, she queers our sense of the ecological body, pointing out that racialised, Indigenous and people with forms of disability are overwhelmingly made to absorb environmental harms over generations. She argues that our bodies are evolving ecologically so that they endure 'toxic substances' in themselves and in the wider ecological system. Toxicity is a 'matter of management of chemicality that works across communities, across populations' (Chen 2023: 7). She proposes that this toxic reality summons 'queer love' as we attend to the wounds of the world in a search for collective and individual forms of healing and caring for human and more-than-human communities. She suggests that 'thinking and feeling with toxicity invites us to revise, once again, the sociality that queer theory has in many ways made possible' (ibid., 207).

As Chen's provocations suggest, queer and crip[8] theory help us to see how our toxic world is breaking down notions of 'normal' bodies, making visible lives at the intersection of multiple oppressions: race, class, gender, disability and sexual orientation. In the face of environmental destruction, we need to embrace differences and otherness of subjects, human and non-human, in ways that harbour mutual respect and care. Queer and crip activists argue that all bodies are deserving of care, but that racialised, queer and disabled bodies are too often excluded from social and political and ecological thought:

> Our beloved and complex Black, Brown, Indigenous, Fat, Queer, Non-binary, Trans Disabled Bodies are as deserving of care and loving tenderness as any other body on the earth. The brown and green lands and the deforested lands, the fresh clean breezes and the stagnant polluted air, the deep unlit seas and the dying coral reef, all parts of our debilitated powerful earth deserve our respect and our care ... We envision an end to corporate fracking and drilling, even as we mourn countless disappearances of kin species. We feel joy in witnessing flower blossoms even through our grief over red or black skies. May we hold each other through our individual struggles and triumphs, our collective transitions, and beyond.
> Sins invalid Statement on Disability Justice. 7 July 2022[9]

Queer artist and activist Leah Piepzna-Samarasinha (2021) writes passionately about the political need for visibility of sick and disabled queer people of colour in environmental survival and justice. She celebrates the survival skills and knowledge of people living with disability. Building on her years of cultural and activist work, she sees people living with illness and disability as leaders in today's and the future's environmental disasters, where survival skills of how to continue despite fatigue, confusion and panic will be needed. She dreams of a movement in which disability justice will lead the way: 'With all of our crazy, adaptive-deviced, loving kinship and commitment to each other, we will leave no one behind as we roll, limp, stim, sign, and move in a million ways towards cocreating the decolonial living future' (Piepzna-Samarasinha 2021: 40).

Vanessa Raditz is co-founder of Queer Ecojustice Project, a media and education collective. Raditz envisages queer and disabled people as providing guidance on how to survive increasingly tenuous lifeworlds. As she wrote with Patty Berne:

> we have to fight for the valuable lives of butterflies, and moss, and elders. Because our lives – and all life – depends on it . . . Even in the moments when we're in pain, when we're uncomfortable, when the task ahead feels overwhelming, and we feel defeated by the sheer scope of everything that's wrong in the world, we don't have to give up on life or on humanity. Queer and trans disabled people know that, because that's how we live. At this moment of climate chaos, we're saying: Welcome to our world. We have some things to teach you if you'll listen, so that we can all survive.
>
> Raditz and Berne 2019: np

Her message is that queer and disabled people are disrupting norms in a world of crisis. They hold valuable and needed skills to create communities that are inclusive and can regenerate and build deep relationships that reconnect human and more-than-others in mind, body and spirit.[10]

Ecofeminism has long recognised that humans are bound in deep connections with more-than-human others in a heteropatriarchal world (Gaard 1993). Since the 1980s ecofeminism has argued for greater attention to interspecies relations and 'how to get on in this Anthropocenic world in more just and caring ways' (Neimanis 2015: 1). While ecofeminism was seen as essentialist and ignored in the 1980s and 1990s (Gaard 2012: 32), it has seen a resurgence since the 2010s. Ecofeminism has taken up an intersectional approach, veering away from white liberal feminism to 'critique of economic imperialism, cultural and ecological colonialism, gender and species oppression' (Gaard 2012: 44). Ecofeminism joins queer and disability studies as it considers how 'sexism, heteronormativity, racism, colonialism, ableism, speciesism, and environmental degradation' intersect (Neimanis 2015: 3).

As part of the resurgence of ecofeminism, veganism has become recognised as a practice and theory that is based on the embodied and material connections with the environment and the maltreatment of animals (Adams 1991: 2012). Vegan feminism is concerned about the structural oppression of animals, criticising the exploitative and violent system around meat consumption as well as scrutinising how humans treat other species and environments. Veganism sees human relations with more-than-human beings as deeply unequal and argues for 'an end to the domination and power' being exerted over both wild and companion animals 'to control their territories, behaviours and freedoms' (Oliver 2024: 33). In an expansive call for an ethics of care based on activism to end animal suffering, vegan feminism 'promotes compassion' for more-than-human others (Oliver 2024: 31) that allows humans to 'reposition our relationship with the environment' (Adams 1991: 140).

As debates around veganism suggest, there are a slew of conundrums in relation to how to change our relations to animals, beginning with modern western cultures that invisiblise animal deaths for food as well as for science. Lynda Korimboccus, writing from the UK, speaks of the 'Peppa Pig paradox' (Korimboccus 2024: 75), where children are on the one hand encouraged to feel affection for animals with visits to zoos and petting farms as well as through animated figures such as the cartoon Peppa Pig,[11] while at the same time they are told to eat up their meat and drink their milk in everyday acts which normalise and hide the violence of slaughterhouses. Such behaviour builds the perception that factory farming and animals are commodities that exist 'for' human benefit (Korimboccus 2024: 76). These writings show how the animal-industrial complex has enormous impact on the lives of more-than-human species, an impact we have normalised as part of the intertwined toxicity of modern economic and ecological relations (Twine 2024).

Black feminist thinking and action on the 'interconnections between social life and social death' are key to understanding the toxicity of our shared embodied ecologies. Jessica Gordon-Nembhard

(2023) underlines Black American women's roles developing co-op ecosystems as part of a 'strategy for liberation'. She argues that black women practice solidarity and cooperative ethical economics as they navigate through the oppressive, exploitative and traumatising effects of capitalism and state violence.

Giovanna Di Chiro, in her writing on toxicity and how it wreaks havoc on the health and reproductive possibilities of the living world (Di Chiro 2010: 210), speaks of how much she has learnt from black women leaders in community-based organisations. In the fight against toxic facilities polluting their and Di Chiro's neighbourhoods they have 'challenged dominant, white male-stream constructions of environmentalism and human-nature relationships'.[12] Like disability justice and queer vegan ecofeminists, black women leaders are actively engaged in the practice of radical hope centred on their reciprocal responsibility to their body, community and life-worlds. Di Chiro shows how interspecies care comes from places and people whose bodies and communities have been 'reviled, neglected, and polluted' (ibid., 200). Di Chiro calls out the gendered, racialised, ableist and heteronormative patterns of mainstream environmentalism and its 'toxic sexism', where feminised bodies are seen as monstrous and queer and crip bodies are cast as 'deviant, impure, or contaminated' (ibid.). She argues that all our lives are entangled with the environment even if we 'imagine our bodies as separate from, unaffected by, and unconnected to our environments' (ibid., 215). Di Chiro quotes biologist, environmentalist and feminist Nancy Langston:

> we're all in this together: the atrazine that gets sprayed on my neighbor's cornfields ends up in the river water, then in the fish, then in the herons and the raccoons that eat the fish – and it also ends up in my breasts, my belly, and my blood. What's out there in wildlife and wild places is also in our bodies.
>
> Nancy Langston, quoted in Di Chiro 2010: 215

These are difficult topics. How to acknowledge our complicity in the marginalising of others, and the impact of our consumerist lifestyles that relies on intoxications of all kinds (Cielemęcka and Åsberg 2019: 105)? As well as reading scholarly and activist texts that speak about the toxic entanglement of human and other bodies in an increasingly degraded and exploited environment, I have found that political and experimental art helps me to grasp emotionally what is human complicity and responsibility for toxic harm in relation to environmental and interspecies care. Art helps us to move into 'speculative dimensions of multispecies worlds' (Pratt 2019: 438) that probe deeper into messy and damaging impacts of environmental change and who deserves to be considered worthy of care.[13]

One of the most engaging speculative artists I have come across is Patrizia Piccinini, an Australian feminist artist who looks at ethical questions around human's responsibility with other species and the more-than-human world in a series of technoscience speculations. Her arresting sculptures and installations present the viewer with 'worlds needy for care and response, worlds full of unsettling but oddly familiar critters who turn out to be simultaneously near kin and alien colonists' (Haraway 2011: 1). Piccinini's art blurs the animate and non-animate, flesh and technology with natural/technical monsters that are cuddly in weird and curious ways. The eerily life-like mannikins are hybrid human, animals, plants and cells creating speculative new worlds where nature and culture are 'tightly knotted in bodies, ecologies, technologies and times' (ibid., 5).

Australian philosopher Susan Pratt, in her discussions of how artists are engaging in speculative acts of care centred on food and entanglements with multispecies others, adds the dimension of radical non-anthropocentric notions of humans as good food for others when we die and return to the Earth. She is inspired by Plumwood's analytic of 'being prey' in her essay 'Eye of the crocodile' (1995) (discussed in

Chapter 3). Plumwood's 'being prey' – of conceiving of oneself in the mouth of a crocodile, challenges human mastery over the food chain and queers what it means to be good food in toxic ecologies. This introduces the multispecies concept of humans as both eater and eaten and expands discussions of care, toxics and multispecies relating. In this move artwork makes visible some of the indirect impacts of toxins and helps articulate different relations mobilised by toxicity and eating.[14] Visual artist Miriam Simun's work interrogates the implications of socio-technical and ecological change. For example, in 'The Lady Cheese Shop' (2013),[15] she displays cheese made from human breast milk, raising questions around the commodification of other mammals and the uneven distribution of toxins to animals in industrial food systems, providing a radical reimagining of life under ecological crisis.

In her discussion of art and food Pratt raises the question about how care for multispecies kin can include understanding how the food chain is being polluted, and how we ourselves are no longer 'good food'. Our bodies are full contaminants from the water we drink, the food we eat and the air we breathe. Our multispecies relations include the microbes within our bodies. We are 'entangled within' (Pratt 2019: 440).

Jae Rhim Lee's art performance pushes the conversation further in her speculative art, the Infinity Burial Suit. Her performance looks at care for interspecies relations after death.[16] She describes herself as 'an artist at the intersection of art, science and culture' (2011). Rhim Lee uses technoscience and art to reconfigure humanity's present and future engagements in permanently toxic worlds as an act of responsibility and care. She argues that we need to take responsibility for the environmental toxins that are stored in our bodies by considering what will happen to the 219 toxic pollutants in our bodies, including preservatives, pesticides and heavy metals like lead and mercury, when we die and our bodies return to the environment.

In the Infinity Burial Project Rhim Lee designs a burial suit that uses mushrooms to decompose and clean toxins in bodies. The dead decomposing body in its suit then delivers nutrients to plant roots, leaving clean compost. She presents the suit as a way for humans to take responsibility for their footprint/burden on the planet.[17] Rhim Lee's work positions human bodies as both live and dead matter. As in life, as in death, humans are part of ecological nourishment for other species and organisms. 'The story passes on to the other life forms you nurture with your death, nurturing those who have nurtured you, in a chain of mutual life-giving' (Plumwood 2004: np, quoted in Pratt, 449). Rhim Lee's burial suit is an example of what Puig de la Bellacasa calls 'more caring affective ecologies' (2017: 219). It is an art project that helps to counter slow violence of pollution as part of a politics of interspecies care. Such art, linked to a feminist politics of care and ethical relations, helps us to speculate on our interspecies entanglements in life and after death.

Conundrums of interspecies care

In this chapter we have taken a journey through feminist texts and actions that are proposing how we can learn and take responsibility for interspecies care. They invite us to take hope in the possibilities still left for our wounded world by paying attention to the compassion of black women activists, queer and disability justice activists, ecofeminists and feminist vegans to consider how our toxic world can produce a new politics and kinship among people and more-than-human beings. Their writings are full of imagination of different possible worlds and offer humbling indications of the dangers in which humanity has placed all life on Earth. Learning from these writings and visual art, we can reconfigure engagements in permanently toxic worlds, and find practices and engagements that involve forms of care for self and human communities which are simultaneously a means of caring for other species.

To return to my brief opening story of interspecies entanglement of my childhood in urban Adelaide in the 1970s, I learnt about the conundrums of caring for animals that could so easily suffer and die due to their capture by humans, however lovingly enacted. We have moved from that simple story to explore more complex issues of ecological embodiment, toxicity, queer theory, wounds of the world and environmental destruction. We have considered the difficulty of expressing love for and our concern at death and loss for/of more-than-human others. The conundrum is that interspecies care is about fear and grief at the extent of loss and death that humans and all beings on our planet are facing (Gruen 2014). In the art of noticing with hope and curiosity we need to make visible the messy embodied entanglements humans have with the more-than-human and recognise what we are losing by failing to embrace an ethics of care for more-than-human others. As Haraway states: 'To care is wet, emotional, messy, and demanding of the best thinking one has ever done' (Haraway 2011: 6).

In Chapter 6 we turn to further inspirational writings and actions, looking at communities of care in the networks of scholars and activists who are building alternatives to mainstream development through post-development practices such as degrowth and community economies.

6

Caring Communities: Building Reciprocity through Degrowth, Community Economies and Radical Care

Unlike the critical stance, which is often suspicious and dismissive, the reparative stance is receptive and hospitable, animated by care for the world and its inhabitants.

J. K. Gibson-Graham 2006: 6.

What we explore in this chapter

Chapter 6 focuses on inspiring communities of scholar activists who see care as a political project that is reparative and helps to build better worlds. It looks at politics that centres care in community building, commoning and radical mobilisations. The opening story is about my experiences engaging in scholar activist communities, taking the example of organising the 8th Degrowth conference. In the second section we turn to the inspiring activities of the Community Economies Research Network (CERN), looking at diverse economies followed by reflections on commoning based on care with more-than-human others. The third section delves into the politics of radical care; popular peasant movements, degrowth communities, international coalitions working for justice for care workers; disability rights activists; queer and transfeminist coalitions.[1]

Section One: *Caring encounters*

Over the years I have been a member of different activist research communities where we practiced collective care as part of our ethics of working together. One such project, 'Women and the Politics of Place', lasted over seven years. I continue to be in touch with most of the participants, though the project ended in the early 2000s. Such projects are part of what I think of as meshworks rather than organised networks. These meshworks thread through my life as loose connections, not bound to any specific institutional arrangement but to a shared commitment to transformative actions around (in my case) gender, environment and social justice.[2]

A meshwork with which I have engaged in the last five years has been the degrowth community. I have engaged in degrowth spaces to give talks on feminism and degrowth for academic and activist communities in the Netherlands, Denmark, Spain and Germany. The most extensive degrowth political project in which I have been involved was the organising collective of the 8th Degrowth Conference. Entitled 'Caring Communities for Radical Change,' it was held as a hybrid event in the Hague during August 2021, as much of Europe came out of lockdown. Care was at the heart of the conference, both practically and thematically. The invitation to join the conference announced: 'care through solidarity and justice' was 'central to degrowth as a collective project promoting sustainable, decolonial, feminist and post-capitalist modes of flourishing'.[3] The core message of degrowth is that 'caring for climate, caring for earth, and caring for people should be at the centre of economic value, not at the margins' (Di Chiro 2019: 306).

It was a complex couple of years as we prepared for the conference. The organising group was intergenerational, a mix of artists, activists, students and professors with varying degrees of engagement in degrowth as a practice. Due to Covid-19 the organising committee, after one face-to-face meeting, operated mostly online. This involved a process of care as we used non-corporate sector software and relied on group members who understood open-source technologies to patiently help the rest of us to navigate unfamiliar IT systems. The weekly meetings held during lockdown were a valuable lifeline to a caring community. We allowed time for self-care as we shared our shock and concern at what was happening in the world. We held out the hope that the conference process itself could change mindsets as we built a caring degrowth community. The original close-knit group expanded rapidly as the conference day grew closer. We moved from an 8-member organising team to a 60-person strong Assembly. Together we learnt to deal with the postponements due to Covid-19, the struggle for funds, and the shared burden of responsibility in holding a 1000-person conference with all the hoops we had to jump through to assure authorities it would be held in Covid-19-safe conditions.

By the time of the conference the Assembly was operating smoothly on principles of care, solidarity, transparency and consensus decision making. The principles were honed through the process of preparing the conference as we challenged norms in relation to age, gender, academic and professional hierarchies. Acting with care is not always easy in groups coming together to work for a specific time bound purpose. Dealing with personal tensions can be time consuming and can feel counterproductive, but we paid attention to tensions as part of the caring political process. The Assembly created lively ways to listen to its members, and to acknowledge all contributions, however small. The 100 volunteers who received free entry to the conference in lieu of pay were fulsomely thanked in public. Whether you were serving lunches, or designing the website or speaking at the opening plenary, everyone was seen as a member of the community.

Key to the process was to use artistic expression as a way to produce knowledge, connection and care. The films, podcasts, drawing, theatre, exhibitions and performances were as much part of the conference as the workshops, lectures and plenaries. Academics who had traditionally dominated degrowth events were encouraged to unlearn their expected position of privilege, to step back and work with different forms of knowledge and to engage in conversations which did not highlight academic knowledge but communication and engagement.

A recent article on collaboration among grassroots organisations and movements working towards ecological sustainability and social justice in Utrecht resonates with my experience. Feola et al. (2025) analyse the challenges of building and sustaining diverse coalitions. The processes they pinpoint include: constructing a collective identity; finding ways to reach agreements on agendas; and barriers related to power asymmetries. Fundamental to movement solidarity organising are trust, commitment and adequate resources, as well as flexible organisational forms. As I also experienced, success rests on 'personal, emotional, institutional, and material connections' and 'decision-making by the people directly impacted by the environmental unsustainability or social injustice' (ibid., 18).

At the Degrowth Conference, held in the long days of the late Dutch summer, there were many levels of connection and engagement. Taking care to be inclusive and ensure wellbeing was paramount: from the diversity in the opening plenaries; to catering for collective meals in different community spaces; to offering forest bathing and participatory art spaces; to holding online panels at times that allowed for international participation. We put together a mega finale in a theatre venue which had hosted The Rolling Stones. It was a decision we could only take a week before, once the municipality agreed the event complied with Covid-19 rules. Age, culture, language, gender, desires, emotions, all bubbled into teeming encounters. It felt like hard work as I collected rubbish, facilitated sessions, handed out drinks, tidied up plates, tried to keep up with all the organisational decisions, met so many varied people. I was grateful that we provided slower, quieter spaces.

One such space was a living sculpture made of mushrooms called the Mycelium Tower, tucked away at the edge of the conference venues. The space attracted not only conference participants but also the neighbours, who joined in convivial conversations around the sculpture, discussing what radical change could mean. Arne Hendriks, a Dutch artist, created the Mycelium Tower using recycled oyster mushroom materials. During the conference participants were invited to harvest the mushrooms and local communities continued to harvest them after the event. The tower was built in a commons garden and provided a quiet space for conversations during the sunny late afternoons. We spoke about what degrowth meant – How do we put care rather than growth at the centre of our daily lives? How do we care for the more-than-human others? Is it possible to have an intergenerational sharing of resources? Can we create safe spaces that are non-violent and inclusive? How can Europeans create caring communities in a globally unequal world? Who is the 'we' that will create change?

The spirit of hope filtered throughout the conference; even if at times it felt overwhelming, it was a creative and exciting space. The main messages of the conference captured in pithy phrases were to 'think positively so you can become part of the change you want to see' – practising prefigurative politics 'to live simply so others might simply live'.

What I learnt from engaging in the organising group was that even if we shared the same goal, to build caring communities meant we had to be aware of diversities. It was important to learn and unlearn our ignorance about those differences, recognising social factors, culture, age and gender. We need to take the time to work through difference if we are to be truly caring. The engagement with the degrowth conference process during Covid-19 opened ways to unsettle major economic narratives. Even if it did not lead to immediate transformations, it did point to the small changes we could make in our everyday lives. Particularly in the European context it meant we had to learn to find ways to take the time to care, such as the caring encounters in the community garden around the Mycelium Tower.

A personal conundrum was how I could best be involved as an older person (by quite some years). My decision was to step aside and be available as a mentor, to support others, and importantly, not to impose my memories and nostalgia for events in which I had been involved over the years. I listened to the younger colleagues balancing care work, precarity and problems of finding livelihoods. I became aware of the stress, mental health and increasing gender violence in their lives during Covid-19. I also heard their stories of strength and resilience in community kitchens, joint childcare arrangements, neighbourly support, experiments in co-creation on and offline as artists worked with academics and activists. I realised I was in a different life moment from them, learning more about the perils of ageing bodies and how to bear the loss of loved ones, but I still felt part of the caring community.

Moving from my personal story of the 8th Degrowth Conference, I now turn to other forms of caring communities which are part of the meshworks around transformative politics: community economies and commoning.

Section Two: *Community economies and commoning*

The Community Economies Research Network (CERN) is a worldwide network of researchers founded by the feminist scholar activists J. K. Gibson-Graham.[4] CERN questions capitalism's position as the all-encompassing signifier of modern economics. They research diverse economies as sites for political and social transformation through collective actions that aim to create more caring sustainable and equitable worlds. Following J. K. Gibson Graham's critique of capitalocentricism (2006), the economy is seen as 'a diverse array of economic relations and practices' including 'non-capitalist relations and enterprises' (Burke and Shear 2014: 134). They 'reclaim the economy as a site of ethical decision-making and practice.... [T]he economy, rather than being seen as "out there" in the stock markets and corporate headquarters of global cities, has been "domesticated", brought down to size and made visible as a site of everyday activities and familiar institutions' (Gibson-Graham and Roelvink 2009: 329). 'Everyday economic activities sustain livelihoods in homes, communities and environments' helping to meet peoples' social, material and emotional needs. Such diverse economies allow 'communities to survive well (rather than just survive) with humans and more-than-human others' (Dombroski et al. 2019: 113).

CERN is operating over generations, space and time. It is an organic network-building community where the insights, care and generosity of J. K. Gibson-Graham are like a pebble thrown into a lake which ripples out to include more and more people and places. CERN's research and engagement with communities are undertaken in solidarity with care and foster hope for reparative actions. They push against academic hierarchies in an open and inclusive sharing of knowledge, in their support of each other and the communities with whom they work. For example, the annual Liviana Conferences are designed to be held online in different time zones so everyone in the network can participate, whether in Australia, New Zealand, Latin America, Europe or Africa. CERN members have collectively produced edited handbooks and books and have a series with Minnesota University Press.[5] The CERN website bristles with information.[6] The network's open and engaged scholarship builds from the embodied participatory research with artists, activists, students, policy makers and communities who seek economic alternatives. Such a pluriversal approach to the production of knowledge about the economy reflects where many of the studies take place, in out-of-the-way places of economically marginal communities in both rural and urban settings.

At the core of CERN, caring practice is to build from encounters that support the wellbeing of communities. The research 'starts where you are' learning with communities about the economy as a site of politics in particular places and regions. My own engagement on the fringes of CERN is indicative of how it is open to include others as a caring research community. By maintaining the network as a 'knowledge commons' (Gibson-Graham et al. 2013: 130), CERN welcomes all people who are interested in learning with them about possibilities for alternative economies.

An ethic of care is central to Community Economies thinking: '[t]he question of how to transform our economies in order to allow human and more than human communities to "survive well together" places care for planetary companions at the heart of our endeavours' (Dombroski, Healy and McKinnon 2018: 99). It is in these ethical negotiations around everyday care practices and care concerns that the strength of the community economies network emerges.[7]

For example, *Take back the economy* (TBTE)[8] (Gibson-Graham et al. 2013) is designed as a tool kit for communities to understand how to engage in local economies. Along with the printed book there is a richly detailed and accessible website which incorporates examples of communities world-wide that are building economies that are socially and environmentally just. TBTE provides 'thinking tools for people who want to start where they are to take back their economies – in countries rich or poor, in neighbourhoods or in nations, as groups or as individuals' (Gibson-Graham et al. 2013, xiv). TBTE encourages the reader to see the economy as something they can understand and engage in locally:

each economy reflects decisions around how to care for and share a commons, what to produce for survival, how to encounter others in the process of surviving well together, how much surplus to produce, how to distribute it, and how to invest it for the future.

ibid., xvii

TBTE provides concrete illustrations of 'alternative economic organizations and practices that are creating socially and environmentally sustainable community economies' (xxii). For example, when discussing how communities can build reciprocal relations, they point to community support groups such as Urban Roots in the US, Wairapa Eco Farms in NZ, Food Connect in Australia and complementary currency networks such as LETs and timebanks in the UK and Australia. TBTE presents economies as centred on 'caring for others and the planet' to meet local economic needs. The picture is a positive one of people maintaining, replenishing and growing natural and cultural communities.

Another inspiring illustration of CERN research is Kelly Dombroski's feminist, postdevelopment and embodied engagement with communities in out-of-the-way places. Her ethnography *Caring for life: A postdevelopment politics of infant hygiene* (2024a) challenges and reworks ways to understand infant care, learning from mothers' and grandmothers' everyday practices of care for infants in Qinghai province, China. She describes the practice of *weisheng* or guarding life as integral to communal wellbeing, where mothers and grandmothers saw their role as protecting the lives of the most vulnerable, including the practice of babies being held out to defecate and urinate freely. She reflects on how she learnt from these practices as she embarked on her own embodied everyday practices of caring for her infants first in China and then with OzNappyfree, an online group of parents based in Australia and Aotearoa, New Zealand, who were learning how to practice nappy-free infant care.

Her approach involved using her own bodily experiences to understand care practices across Chinese and western regions. She writes about how paying attention to what was happening in her body helped her unlearn her assumptions and biases around infant care. As she explains, 'By immersing myself in the daily lives and practices of these communities and paying attention to when I felt moments of "awkward engagement" present in my body, I was able to gain a deeper, more nuanced understanding of caregiving methods and spaces in China's far west' (2024b: np). Her research on nappy/diaper-free hygiene practices is an example of postdevelopment research which offers 'the potential for rethinking hygiene and sanitation in the Western world' (ibid.). She moves across scales from intimate practice of community-based infant care to larger issues such as waste and strategies for sustainable environmental health. The OzNappyFree online community learnt alternative hygienic sustainable practices from communities in rural China. This infant health management can be viewed in the context of larger questions of sanitation infrastructures enforced by government and industry norms. She shows how caring communities of practice can enact alternative ways of raising an infant which are less environmentally damaging, less resource-intensive and waste-producing. Dombroski illustrates how sustaining and maintaining economies in the everyday work of women caring for infants have wider implications for humanity and the planet.

The focus of Dombroski's work on infant health is an example of the original, even quirky, scholarship that emerges from CERN's research with communities that are supporting and constructing economies and ecologies from diverse perspectives outside of mainstream economic analysis. CERN's studies are infused by socio-ecological realities that are often not noticed in mainstream economic narratives. What CERN shows is how communities negotiate and sustain relations as part of economic and social everyday life. In this approach, CERN makes visible ways of being in the world that confirm the existence and possibilities of alternative economics, societies and ecologies (Burke and Shear 2014: 129).

The relationships, practices and initiatives found in grassroots solidarity movements for climate justice, fair trade activism, community networks of food solidarity, slow food, transition towns and politicised research methodologies are the focus of CERN's interest (ibid., 135). These alternative economic institutions are bound by solidarity and mutual relations and the economy is analysed as 'a fundamentally ethical sphere of socio-ecological relations' (ibid.). For example, Cristina Grasseni's study on Italian alternative food networks – *Gruppi di Acquisto Solidale* G.A.S. – explores changes in local economies through social networks that change consumer awareness and support local food growers. Grasseni describes how economic relations based on trust between consumer and producer are built through the direct and collective transactions of G.A.S. building-scale economies of trust. During the earthquakes in L'Aquila (in 2009) and Modena (in 2011), consumers supported farmers by buying and selling damaged food products before they spoiled (Grasseni 2014: 182). Ten years after her CERN study, G.A.S. groups can be found in most regions in Italy, including where I live in Lazio, operating via local assemblies based on solidarity reflecting local relationships that have evolved, eschewing mainstream market practices and trade union hierarchy of formal delegations or elected representatives.

The commoning of resources, knowledge and skills is one of the key strategies of community economies. Through the practice of commoning, communities ensure that access to collective goods is shared, and all members of the community see themselves as not only using and benefiting but also as caring and responsible for goods and produce held in common. Commoning is also a politicised practice of care where communities reclaim and reappropriate local environmental resources.

I use the term commoning to refer to the political process of building community via collective care as a process of transformation and change (Singh 2018; Sato and Soto Alarcón 2019). The practice of commoning encompasses the economic social relations built in the networks and practices organised around solidarity, collectivity, cooperation, self-governance and horizontal sharing of power (Federici and Caffentzis 2014; De Angelis 2017). A 'commoning-community' – a community taking care of and responsibility for a common – is constituted through the process of negotiating 'access, use, benefit, care and responsibility' (Gibson-Graham et al. 2016: 196).

Commoning involves not only practices of care for communities of people, but also for more-than-humans (García-López et al. 2021; Singh 2018, 2013). Neera Singh, in her studies of communal care for the forest, describes how people are brought together through their practices of care for the environment, where social relations are 'inseparable from relations to nature' (García-Lopez et al. 2021: 1201). Silvia Federici describes commoning as 'a quality of relations, a principle of cooperation and of responsibility to each other and to the earth, the forests, the seas, the animals' (Federici 2014: 228–229, quoted in Garcia Lopez et al. 2021: 1206–1207).[9] Commoning as a transformative practice of care in 'spaces of creativity and social reproduction' (Clement et al. 2019: 1) becomes an alternative way of doing politics, 'of imagining and enacting pluriversal, postcapitalist worlds that challenge human exceptionalism and bounded individualism' (Singh 2022: 84–85). It is about responsibility to care for all beings – humans and nonhumans – as part of a 'covenant of reciprocity' (Kimmerer 2013).

Dombroski's research on OzNappyFree collective can be understood as a practice of commoning. Members of the collective are caring for their infant members, collectively engaging in hygiene practices as 'a way of caring for ecologies by reducing the flow of household waste, benefiting human and more-than-human communities in the process. . . . OzNappyFree's care-work around the waste stream, infant and parent attachment and communication' (Dombroski 2024a; Dombroski et al. 2016).

CERN (and WEGO) members Nanako Nakamura and Chizu Sato (2023), in their study of *kokorozashi* – community-based economic practices of older women in depopulating rural Shizuoka, Japan – describe how older women have rebuilt communities together to find collective wellbeing. Their collective S*uisha* has diversified its food businesses to produce soba noodles for local markets, hosting farm workshops and ecotourism. In these commoning activities older women are building community through their care for each other and the environment. Their everyday practice of commoning includes taking time to support each other's ageing processes, creating communal ethics based on place-based solidarity, and sharing skills and knowledge.

Sato, writing with Jozelin Maria Soto Alarcón, presents another case of commoning in a women-led cooperative in rural Mexico, which they describe as place-based multispecies commoning practices of care (Sato and Soto Alarcon 2019). The Mexican peasant women reshaped their community in response to men's outmigration from the area to find paid work. This resulted in more work for women as they assumed responsibilities for the family lands and crops as well as households. The women turned to agaves to reappropriate available resources, creating a commoning community which cared for their families, the agaves and the worms, ants and insects with which they shared the land (ibid., 50). Their local language of *Otomi* was revived in the commoning process to incorporate traditional knowledge of agaves, bringing a new sense of belonging to the communities in the region (ibid., 53). In addition, the women's community nurtured common property and practices, providing financial and other social support (ibid., 54). The tasks, or *faena*, they did together were based on reciprocal care and responsibilities from childcare to support for agave-related farming activities (ibid., 55).

Other studies on commoning include *Teis CF*, a community forest group based in Galicia, Spain, which resisted the introduction of tree species of eucalyptus and acacia (Nieto-Romero et al. 2023: 275). Commoning in this case was focused on care for the forest's health. Group members describe how the forest is 'a living being', part of their shared life story, a place to rest and enjoy life, their 'playground' (ibid., 277). Their sense of belonging as a community was shaped by their caring for the forest's ecosystem. As custodians of the forest *Teis CF* saved trees, cared for plants and rescued harmed animals (ibid., 279–280). The group's political resistance to the introduced species grew out of 'lived-in and embodied community practice' and was part of their 'reciprocal restoration' practices of care among these forest 'commoners' (ibid., 282).

A final example of commoning is from Miriam Tola's study (2017) of commons emerging around a ruined lake in the periphery of Rome, which had been poisoned decades earlier by a rayon factory. She describes the 'impure and messy commons that strives to persist in an urban context marked by the increasing precarity of labour and livelihood' (Tola 2017: 196). Tola shows how the commons is an interplay of many kinds of beings, not all of which are human, as she explores how organisational forms bring together geological and ecological forces and provide the conditions for the making of a commons. The neighbourhood and its environs were left to decline for decades after the factory was closed in the 1950s. The attempt by government and local enterprise to revive the area in the 1990s with plans for a commercial centre was fiercely contested by locals and scholar activists, who pushed instead for a public park which acknowledged the toxic history of the area, or what Tola calls its 'eco-memory'. In conversations with older residents who lived in the area, a collective of activists worked with ecologists, engineers and botanists to revive the natural environment around the polluted lake and monitor the area's rich biodiversity. This process of commoning formed the *Forum Parco delle Energie*, which petitioned the local government to recognise the lake as a public domain. The community collective was successful in building an urban ecosystem out of the toxic history of the area, with the lake at its centre (ibid., 210). Tola describes this commoning as a political project of a 'rebel lake' which 'manages to live despite capitalism' (ibid., 211).

Tola sees care as 'the ability to keep life alive', but one that is 'an increasingly conflictual practice'. Care is the radical struggle to push back the necropolitical management of lives, which leads to the neglect of human and more-than-human bodies in an increasingly toxic life on Earth. In her analysis Tola gives agency to the lake as a prime actor in the mobilisation rather than just a resource, an example of 'being-in-common': 'Quietly, the lake, whose waters continue to move and flow, began to exert its force of attraction on the many who learned to care for its existence' (ibid., 208). She speaks of ecomemory which is part of the landscape. I visited this area some years back with my younger daughter on a school excursion where we were taken to see the bird life on the lake, a museum in the remains of the factory and heard the residents speak with pride of the recovery of the lake and their community.

Toba's study is an example of what is becoming a flourishing research area on commoning and communities around water flows throughout the world. For example, the collection by Zwarteveen et al. looks at how groundwater care in India, Morocco, Algeria and Peru is 'embedded in cosmologies that emphasize mutuality and conviviality' as 'communities adapt to the changing circumstances crafting new institutions and infrastructures in processes of commoning' (Zwarteveen et al. 2024: 388). In another study of ecomemory around rivers, Elizabeth Day (2022) reflects on Parramatta River in New South Wales, Australia: 'It is a place still alive with the violence of our colonial history . . . Parramatta was a place of meeting of freshwater and salt-water Aboriginal groups and has a vast history' (Day 2022: 188). Her art visually engages with past pain of colonial violence continued in the institutions that are found along the banks of the Parramatta River associated with punishment, mental health services and migrant services (ibid., 192).

Section Three: *Radical care*

In the final section of this chapter, we explore radical care, where caring is an ethically and politically charged practice (Puig de la Bella Casa 2011). I am interested here in the radical care where the physical and emotional wellbeing of people is central to political transformation. Radical care 'offers visceral, material, and emotional' support to 'selves, communities, and social worlds' (Hobart and Kneese 2020: 2) in groups that share reciprocal relations and collaboration in response to profound neglect and crises (Hobart and Kneese 2020; Reese and Johnson 2022; Edelman 2020).

As we saw in Chapter 2, Manuela Zechner is a fierce advocate for radical care, which begins with human entanglement with all living beings and ecosystems.[10] Zechner sees the starting point for radical care politics as our collective shared vulnerability, economic and ecological precarity in fracturing fragile life-worlds. Zechner points to the world's sacrifice zones, where 'communities, ecosystems, care networks, bodies and lives' live in the ruins of colonialism and capitalism. For her our ecological crisis is due to a 'deep impasse of care (Zechner 2022: np). She argues that in the face of the extractivism and waste of capitalist political economic and colonial systems, it is a political necessity to revalue life through the recognition of our shared vulnerability and need for care. Practising radical care allows us to draw 'on our collective strength and resistance, to sustain lives and worlds in the fight for our interdependence' (ibid.).

Zechner points to current practices of radical care: the 'utopian-experimental work, traditional communities, and technologies (think peasants, Indigenous people), and defensive struggles at the level of territory (think land rights, environmental defenders) and labour (think workers in industrial agriculture)' (ibid.). Strategies such as commoning enable the cultivation of life systems through 'ecological municipalism, transition towns, land defense and habitat protection, community farming and peasant struggle, squatting and collective infrastructure building' (ibid). She asks that we start from where we live and what we live from to foster collective trust and care by acknowledging our 'mutual vulnerability'. The practice or politics of care will lead to 'radical, sustainable, and just ways out of our multiple intertwined crises' (ibid.).

Following Zechner's impetus, we now look at the webs of radical care in degrowth, popular peasant movements, Indigenous and radical feminist struggles, disability and queer feminist activism.

In degrowth, as the opening story of the chapter shows, care is fundamental to degrowth's goal of building radical alternatives which foster collective and welcoming spaces for healing and reconnecting while disrupting narratives of growth and dismantling racialised economic narratives. Degrowth builds on principles that include 'care, sharing, autonomy, solidarity, justice, democracy, and conviviality' (Akbulut 2021: 99). Degrowth aims to integrate caring commoning practices in everyday lives – changing people's relations to food, energy, housing and care, to forge moral and material worlds that prioritise wellbeing, equity and sustainability. This requires a radical embodying of deep change that allows for connections with others and builds community, challenging the primacy of the individual western-self (Kaul et al. 2022). Degrowth sees care as political – 'caring for each other' can produce 'radical hope-infused democratic movements around the world passionately building earth-friendly, subsistence economies for all' (Di Chiro 2019: 310). Such radical care means fighting to end structural racism and inequality, recalling that 'care is profoundly present for those performing its labor and – not uncoincidentally – those most easily overlooked by the politically and socially privileged' (Hobart and Kneese 2020: 7–8). Degrowth is a call 'to break with economic growth as a societal goal and to oppose the automatic association of growth with better outcomes' (Akbulut 2021: 98). There is an explicit effort to connect with the plurality of visions and cosmologies that challenge the hegemony of growth and development in the search for living well (ibid., 100).

La Via Campesina (LVC) is a global popular peasant movement that values social reproduction and the care work of women. LVC has alliances in eighty-one countries, which work to defend peasant agriculture, food sovereignty, the struggle for land, justice and equality, and to eradicate gender discrimination and violence.[11] Over the years LVC has held five international women's conferences or assemblies to ensure that women's work is valued and supported and that peasant women's work on the front line of care work is not taken for granted in the LVC campaigns and mobilisations (LVC 2021). These international meetings have built radical care into peasant and popular feminism to support women's fight for autonomy, social transformation and for food sovereignty, promoting agroecology that ends production with agrotoxics. The fight to end gender-based violence is also part of LVC's fight to end structural unequal relations. LVC sees feminism as a collective process, where women are bound in their fight to take back their body-territories as women produce and reproduce life and culture.

A vibrant Nicaraguan example of popular peasant feminism is FEM, described by feminist activist scholar Ana Victoria Portocarrero Lacayo (2024). Through FEM's practices of radical care, the peasant women sustain themselves and their livelihoods, fending off damages to their seeds, crops and community by climate change, economic insecurity and an increasingly oppressive political regime. Portocarrero Lacayo describes how working together in the fields and in educational spaces, FEM practice radical self-care and community care, valuing their work inside and outside the home and pooling knowledge on agroecological techniques. As a member of the FEM collective states, their radical care for body-territory as they work the fields together using the seeds they have collected and saved is also driven by the political will to

> the fight for the land, for our native seeds, against climate change. We fight for a peasantry that is aware of the tragedy that is happening in their country, of the destruction of nature by the markets, by the invasion of multinationals. We are fighting for a peasantry that is aware of the enormous damage being caused by the agri-food system, which is expressed here in our communities and in our bodies.
>
> Quoted in Portocarrero Lacayo 2024: 5

As well as care for the seeds and land, they also take part in care for each other, supporting strategies to resist physical and sexual violence (ibid., 12). Portocarrero Lacayo shows how FEM's everyday practices are informed by an ethics of care based on traditional knowledge of their farming practices and as women resisting patriarchal and economic violence. In the difficult economic and political context of Nicaragua, peasant women taking care of their bodies and land is a radical act.

Another example of radical care by economically and socially marginalised women who face deep and ongoing oppression is the Aboriginal and Torres Strait Islander Social Justice Wiyi Yani U Thangani Commission for First Nations gender justice and equality in Australia. The commission builds on the voices of Aboriginal and Torres Strait Islander women led by the Aboriginal and Torres Strait Islander Social Justice Commissioner, June Oscar.[12]

The commission's report 'Caring about Care: Wiyi Yani U Thangani' (2023) advocates for the recognition and value of Indigenous women's care work (Klein et al. 2023). It details the care work of 102 women from remote communities and marginalised urban areas in the ACT, Central Australia, Cape York, East Kimberley and Greater Sydney. The policy message of the report is that women's unpaid care is undervalued, unrecognised and requires more support.

The deep insight of the report is due to its wealth of interviews, which show the richness and complexity of care work undertaken mostly by women in the Aboriginal and Torres Strait Islander communities. The women's care work is materially and emotionally vital. It ensures cultural ties, identity, autonomy and health, and the socio-political, cultural, economic and physical and emotional wellbeing of Indigenous peoples (ibid., 18). Care work involves the day-to-day care of children and the elderly, as well as support for family members in the face of settler-induced trauma, violence, state incarceration and the removal of children by the state.

Care in this difficult context is a radical and creative labour of resistance, growth and possibility. Indigenous women's unpaid care labour is at the forefront of struggles against oppressive settler colonial structures. The women's care loads are heavy, much heavier than other groups of women in Australia, and are determined by historic and ongoing colonisation. The women's stories show how caring is a source of strength and courage that is passed down generations. Care is understood as part of each community's 'social glue'. It is the 'web of caregiving' that grows through relations of reciprocity that enable communities to survive (ibid., 57). Women speak about drawing strength from their roles caring for country and culture, including the time taken to pass down knowledge of country (ibid., 58).

In a composite quote from the report, three women from the East Kimberly region explain the importance of Care for Country:

> Well, care for me as an Indigenous person is not just caring for your family, it's caring for your Country ... [Care of Country] is automatically in our, in our blood... Going back to Country and that, that's, that's a really big part for healing as well for Aboriginal people. Like sometimes, like when we live in town, um, your spirit is not there. Your spirit is out there on your Country. So when you go out your Country, you can feel the difference between town and the Country because the, the Country, it will welcome you back in. . . . So country cares for you. Not just you care for it.
>
> ibid., 74

The many interviews provide a vivid sense of how women are holding together complex blended, separated and intergenerational families and communities which have been severely damaged by colonisation's impacts (ibid., 88). Women are dealing with financial struggle and structural marginalisation and intergenerational trauma (ibid., 61). Though exhausting, it is about resistance and radical refusal. As one participant stated:

> I would consider my activism a level of care for my culture because it's a responsibility that I carry to nurture my culture, and what that looks like in the 21st century in a country that is illegally occupied. There is an enormous level of care for my community in that because it's not easy to put yourself out in that space open to scrutiny and to be knocked down by government to be knocked down by even your own mob. I think there is care in our activism. Like our activism comes from a place of love, it comes from a place of survival and wanting to continue our culture.
>
> ibid., 36

The document provides evidence for a different approach to care work that 'elevates Indigenous women's voices, centres and celebrates their care. Far from being peripheral to the economy, what Indigenous women have shown is that care underpins everything. It is a way of life and is essential to the flourishing of human societies. Care is at the heart of any economic system, and the monetised part of the economy cannot be sustained without the underpinning care of Country, culture and people' (ibid., 119).

Valuing care is similarly at the centre of the Global Strike for Women (GWS), a global activist campaign that advocates for a care income. The website declares: 'Mothers and other carers, of every gender, are entitled to a living wage, a Care Income – in cash, land, non-polluting technology – for their caring work for people and planet.'[13] GWS evolved from the International Wages for Housework Campaign started by Selma James in the US in 1972, which argued for payment for care work instead of military spending with the slogan 'Invest in Caring, Not Killing'.

GWS radical campaigns push to end power relations through advocating anti-sexism, anti-racism, anti-deportation and health and environmental justice working with mothers and other carers, women with disabilities, queer women, rape survivors, sex workers and domestic workers. The movement has taken many forms shaped by the autonomous organisations of women of colour, queer women, sex workers, single mothers and women with disabilities within it. GWS contributes to the campaigns of these different coalitions, ranging from the farm workers movement in rural India to Black Lives Matter and the Degrowth movement.[14]

Working with GWS is the Just Transition and Care initiative JTCI,[15] a joint collaboration of the research centre at the University of Santiago de Compostela, Spain, Colorado University USA and UNRISD. JTCI brings care work to the larger Just Transitions coalition of labour and environmental justice organisations that look at climate and ecological transition policies from the perspective of social inequality. The initiative looks at domestic and community caregiving including subsistence food provisioning, health care and environmental care in urban and rural environments, on the land and in other earth-systems. JTCI brings the knowledge and vision of care workers to push for a shift from 'a care-less to a care-full economic system, expanding human rights toward the inclusion of a right to adequate care, to safety from the risks associated with ongoing climate and environmental changes, and to a healthy environment for working class, peasant and Indigenous populations' (Just Transitions 2024: np).

Radical care, as we discussed in Chapter 5, is at the heart of disability justice; what Piepzna-Samarasinha (2018), writing from her bed, describes as 'wild experiments with collective access and care' (Piepzna-Samarasinha 2018: 10). Reflecting with 'broken beautiful wisdom' she asks: 'What does it mean to shift our ideas of access and care (whether it's disability, childcare, economic access, or many more) from an individual chore, an unfortunate cost of having an unfortunate body, to a collective responsibility that's maybe even deeply joyful?' (ibid., 16). Radical care in Piepzna-Samarasinha's words and action becomes 'love work of collective care that lifts us instead of abandons us, that grapples with all the deep ways in which care is complicated' (ibid). The practice of care in her writing is about the politics of autonomy and dignity that recognises the care by marginalised groups as powerful. These emergent resilient networks of care enable people with disabilities 'to care for ourselves and each other for a long time (ibid.) and they need to be at the forefront of transitions to justice'.

As Piepzna-Samarsinha shows, the notion of radical care is about resistance, surviving and creating a liveable life. Care is about struggle, survival and change. Transfeminist scholar Ilenia Iengo writes of her engagement in southern Italy of 'transfeminist care commons', where communities sustain 'bodily autonomy and community interdependency to confront and subvert neoliberal, capitalist, extractivist and patriarchal relations' (Iengo 2025). She describes how ground-up care networks formed around anti-violence centres and community health clinics for women and LGBTQI+ people particularly during Covid-19, which led to further political engagement (ibid.). Such activities are linked to *Non Una di Meno*, an Italian campaign to end male violence against women, the violence of heteronormativity, precarious labour, racism and the European regimes of border control. In their 2022 public statement 'Life Beyond the Pandemic' they point to the nexus between social and ecological reproduction. They declare:

> We need to rethink our life in common, bringing down once and for all the violence of the neoliberal model. . . . Caring, or the ability to keep life alive, becomes an increasingly conflictual practice: to care is to struggle against the necropolitical management of lives, and to struggle is to care for the redistribution of life on Earth.
>
> *Non Una di Meno* 2022: np

Iengo (ibid.) describes how activist networks and social centres in Naples rallied together to provide essential food, sanitary products and meals to disabled, racialised, older and homeless people, providing forms of care infrastructure that sustained life and, in the process, provided the space for political action that demanded more public support for health, rent and income. 'To fight *for* and *with* care means supporting the struggles for universal access to public health, wealth and schools; the struggles against police and state violence; the struggles against the exploitation of communities, common lands and resources' (*Non Una Di Meno* 2020: np).

Elija Adiv Edelman's studies on queer and trans coalitions such as the DC Trans Coalition (DCTC) in Washington underlines the radical importance of care for trans people who live a 'diverse and complex multitude of expressions and identities' (Edelman 2020: 113). Edelman argues that trans coalitions provide 'a kind of care that defies conventional descriptions' because 'life making in trans coalitional spaces may very well coexist within spaces heavily marked by death and loss' and it is 'through the messy and frequently traumatic incoherence of death and loss that we experience the full potential of radical care' (ibid., 111–112). Edelman proposes that an ethics of radical care is at the heart of a radical trans politics. The centrality of radical care is about ways of coping with 'the disturbingly high rates of assault and harassment' and health crises, including denial of medical care experienced by trans persons and mental health issues – including a high rate of attempted suicide (ibid., 115–117). Edelman speaks of coalitions as 'radical forms of care' where radical trans politics and activism 'brings people together, as it acknowledges the pain and difficulties trans persons experience (ibid., 125). Such frameworks of radical care call for a rethinking of care processes to acknowledge that not all bodies, spaces and lives fit a normative framing of rights and politics.[16]

To complete this survey of forms of radical care there are also feminist art and architectural projects which position care as an 'intended urgent and necessary platform . . . to potentially craft a more hopeful future' (Phillips 2022: 268). Elke Krasny (whose work we discussed in Chapter 2) highlights through her curation work how 'care is a radical practice for social transformation' (ibid., 274). In 2020 Krasny curated with Helena Reckitt an art project 'On Caring' to show how the pandemic exposed society's reliance on care work (ibid., 270). Such public art projects open spaces for 'dialogues *about care*, who and what we care for, as well as instigate *acts of care* for others, the environment and all living matter' (Hayes 2022: 227, italics in the original).[17] Radically forming practices of care in public spaces is also the subject of Krazny's edited book with Angelika Fitz on *Critical care: Architecture and urbanism for a broken planet* (2019). Tronto in her essay for the book proposes that 'we need an architecture of care that instead of thinking of buildings as things, thinking of them in relationships with ongoing environments, people, flora and fauna . . . we need an architecture that fulfils the basic task of sharing responsibilities of caring for our world . . . sensitive to the values of repair, of preservation of maintaining all forms of life and the planet itself' (Tronto 2019: 28). As this observation by Tronto suggests, a feminist-inspired, relational, critical care approach could transform architectural practices towards restorative ecologies in response to crises of disasters such as flooding and fires that we face now and in the future.

Conundrums of radical care

What are the conundrums around feminist politics that centres care in community building, commoning and radical mobilisations? Is the call to care a romanticisation complicit in the maintaining of a fundamentally oppressive system, or is the call to care a way to mobilise and break through oppressions?

Feminist theorist Michelle Murphy (2015)[18] aims to unsettle care at the centre of feminist writing and practice as she questions feminist mobilisations of care. She cautions that care is too complex to be easily harnessed in calls for political transformation. She argues that feminist practice and theory often skip the structural histories and arrangements of power that work through feminist good intentions in their appeal to care: 'there is an ongoing temptation within feminist scholarship to view positive affect and care as a route to emancipated science and alternative knowledge-making without critically examining the ways positive feelings, sympathy, and other forms of attachment can work with and through the grain of hegemonic structures, rather than against them' (ibid., 720).

She asks that critical feminist theory and practices be more 'accountable to the economic, racialized, and colonial entanglements of both science and feminism' (ibid., 721). She warns against 'conflating care with affection and attachment' and falling into the 'romantic temptation' that 'positive feeling' is a 'political good' disconnected from geopolitical contexts (ibid., 724).

Murphy sees 'matters of care' as violently entangled in 'development projects, public health practices, labor stratigraphies, family planning practices, humanitarian interventions, pedagogy, family formations' (ibid., 724). Provocatively she argues that care can be a form of racialised violence because it is threaded throughout history in 'racialized and transnational itineraries of "intimacy" and "care" in processes of immigration, citizenship, family law, sex work, tourism' (ibid.). She warns that feminist projects of care can be complicit with dominant economic and political systems if they claim to be reparative and working towards a better world. Such projects can be 'folded into a larger anti-colonial rearrangement of the uneasy work of fostering life' (ibid., 725). In short, Murphy sees the appeal to care as a driving force for mobilisation as delusional.

I would argue instead that the stories in this chapter are inspirational and grounded. What they show is that care is embedded in powerful material and embodied relations and operates in political projects that engage people in ways that make the world a better place. They offer us examples of what is already happening in different communities and places where experimentation and improvisation flourish as means of survival. The world is in deep trouble, even if it is hard to find ways to talk about it, and diverse economic practices show ways forward, based on nurturing others rather than mastery (Hine 2023). The examples in this chapter show how sharing experiences provides knowledge of some non-capitalist paths that are worth taking. As Gibson-Graham and Dombroski state eloquently:

> Transforming the economy is a project of shifting subjectivities – our sense of selves as agents and actors. It is a project of shifting language – moving towards languages of possibility and care. It is a project of developing capacity for collective action through multiple means. And it is a project of finding the joy in collective action, where we act because acting is the next right thing to do, not because we necessarily know how it will turn out.
>
> Dombroski and Gibson-Graham 2025: np[19]

Degrowth, community economies and radical care communities invite us to consider ways to work in reciprocal relations in encounters that share commons and enhance wellbeing for humans and more-than-humans now and into the future (Gibson-Graham and Dombroski 2020: 19). Degrowth repositions economic imperatives by 'invoking questions of production for whom, of what, under what conditions, and with which consequences echo[ing] the nodes of ethical-political decision-making unearthed by the community economies framework' (Akbulut 2021: 101). These visions are based on care as sustaining (human and more-than-human) life that challenges Global North epistemological privilege and points to the

Global North's responsibilities to degrow to allow others more space to live (Akbulut 2024: np).

As Rebecca Solnit (2024) points out, we act with care when we see crisis as offering hope. We need to recognise the uncertainty of the future, 'navigate through despair' and find the 'possibilities of bringing together the many ways people can and do work together' (Dombroski and Gibson-Graham 2025: np). In doing so we reject crisis-fuelled capitalist techno-managerialism and with hope, find ways to act together in solidarity. Coming together to find strategies for alternatives is more crucial than ever today in the wake of today's cuts to education and development emboldened by Trump's destructive acts destroying ecologies, economies, societies and the academy.

In the final chapter of the book, I discuss what these different approaches and debates around care mean for critical development in theory and practice and the importance of holding space for hope rather than despair. I share stories from my experience of teaching and then reflect on ethically aware development 'otherwise' teaching that takes care as an invitation to foster cross-cultural understandings of human and more-than-human wellbeing. I argue that development discourse needs to connect much more deeply with care in order to challenge and change destructive economic and environmental practices of capitalist development processes.

Connecting with Care: Pedagogies for Transformation

To understand the world is to change it. As a performative practice, academic research is activism; it participates in bringing new realities into being.

J. K. Gibson-Graham and G. Roelvink 2009: 342.

What we explore in this chapter

This chapter begins with reflections on my experiences of teaching with care as a pedagogical approach. I start with a story of a recent conversation with two former students. Section Two looks at ethically aware teaching as part of critical development practice, taking examples from friends and colleagues who are teaching students to find ways to repair and reconnect life-worlds. The final section looks at how critical development in theory and practice should be repositioned to connect more deeply to care to address the violence of racism, speciesism, capitalism, imperialism and patriarchy.

Section One: *Teaching with care*

On a chilly November morning I was sitting in an elegant courtyard in The Hague, drinking coffee and thoroughly enjoying a conversation with two former ISS students, now friends for several years. Our conversation had begun by sharing our different assessments of the savage right turn in US and Dutch politics leading to massive cuts to education, human rights, LGBTQ and gender programmes. I was squelching the rumours circulating that the building where my institute was located, the old post office, was about to be sold. They were informing me how their non-government organisations (NGOs) were dealing with impending cuts, the need to reorganise, change strategies and resist co-optation. They were adamant that International NGOs (INGOS) were as much to blame as governments for the dire situation; both had failed to deliver on the promises for human rights. Listening to their stories, I was impressed by their political savvy and capabilities. I felt compelled to ask, 'Wouldn't it be better that they were back home fighting inside their governments, rather than dealing with the precarity and prejudice in this cold northern city where they experienced racism and prejudice?' They both turned to me with a look of surprise. What a blunder I thought: they could not be open about their sexuality nor live as a couple back home. But that was not what concerned them. Rather, they explained, they could exercise greater power as activists in the Global North than in the Global South. Changing prejudice around human rights issues required international pressure. As Global South activists working in local organisations in Europe, they were compensated fairly and they could ensure direct links with local groups and apply pressure on governments and INGOs. Even given the worsening funding situation, they had more potential to change the discourse around gender, human rights and LGBTQI+ issues here than in their countries, where they would be swallowed up in bureaucracy or silenced or worse. They wanted to be inside the belly of the beast, fighting and negotiating where they could be the most disruptive and the most effectively heard, speaking to power.

There are many conundrums of teaching in a critical international development in higher education. I am connecting with students from around the world, for a brief heady moment, who know far better than I do the realities of what international development has meant in their country. Yet I am expected to be the expert. I present them with questions whereas many students come expecting applicable practices and blueprints for change. I see successful teaching as when students think of the questions *with* me, and we learn to connect across generations and cultures. We listen to different points of view, building a reciprocal relationship which allows us to see the cracks in the system in order to resist and push for change.

When it is possible to cross barriers of age, culture and language, education becomes a caring, learning process. Over the years I have learnt to recognise the moment when a student realises they can cross the line. It can be when they ask a question in a lecture, share a quiet moment in my room, or a chance encounter out of the classroom or over a coffee.[1] Perhaps the hardest thing for me is that I cannot force that moment. I am wistful about the students in whom I saw the possibility of connection, but it didn't materialise. When it does happen, it can be life affirming for us both. I am deeply touched when I hear from students about how their connection with me at ISS impacted and changed their lives and careers. I have also learnt not to care when students disappear from my life as our connection fades into the past along with their ISS experience, even if news might occasionally surface via social media.

I end this introduction with another personal story that illustrates pedagogies of care. As I mentioned in Chapter 1, teaching development studies is about taking risks to disrupt dominant narratives that knowledge is about expertise, neutrality, facts and figures which a university education will impart. Emotions and affect are not traditionally seen as part of academic learning. In the MA and university college classes I have taught on political ecology, I have invited students to confront their fears and concerns around climate change, biocides, failings of democracies and deepening economic inequalities. One of the pedagogical tools I use is to visualise their thoughts through painting, drawing, collages or zines. Using creative visual representation allows students to promote ecological imaginaries. Such pedagogies break down knowledge hierarchies and open possibilities to connect with others (Harcourt 2019). By collectively sharing the emotional impact of climate and environmental crisis in their drawings and collages, students become more open to share the impact of environmental change in their lives and to consider in what ways they can respond. In one session I invite students to draw how they imagine socio-natural relations in 2063. I have been enthralled by their utopian imaginaries of interspecies co-habitation and quirky forms of flourishing ecodiversity. I have also been taken aback at dystopic drawings of life-worlds ruled by extreme weather conditions, where the few surviving humans live in hyper-tech fort-like structures to keep out monster insects that have adapted to arid or flooded landscapes.

Circling back to the conversation with my two friends, in my years of teaching I have become aware of how important it is to make sure students know that if academic discourse is to be transformative, it must be linked to processes of political change which are happening outside the university. As my friends described it to me, they bring theory and practice together in their NGO trainings and workshops on sexuality and gender. They engage in a caring process of reciprocal learning as they use their knowledge to push for audacious strategies that can disrupt and bring about change. My continuing connection with such students is what bell hooks calls 'engaged pedagogy' (hooks 1994) – a connection that emerges in the classroom but travels across a lifetime. Even if students can find such ways of teaching unsettling at the time, when over the years they return into your life to share their stories, as a teacher you feel both the responsibilities and the possibilities of the classroom.[2]

This can happen in various ways. As one of the friends told me they were so inspired by the conversations we had on the politics of care and the need for new imaginaries, they brought that learning into a sideline panel for LGBTQI+ rights they organised at the UN High-Level Political Forum in July 2024 called 'A Queer Future of Care'. The session was based on imaginaries and storytelling about futures of care from Armenia, Kenya, Namibia, Nepal, Peru, Uganda and Zimbabwe. The drag queen Envy Peru lip synched to Michael Jackson's 'Earth Song' as a form of self-expression and political activism that 'contributes to diversity and inclusivity and embodies the concept: Leave no one behind'.[3] As my friend stated, in a playful but serious comment, they held such an event in the UN because 'we cannot afford half-arsed feminism'.

Section Two: *Careful disruptions*

I have learnt how to teach with care by learning from colleagues how to acknowledge my own vulnerability, pain and anger, and from that position, be able to care enough to engage with students on ways to repair our broken world. By co-teaching, or by sharing syllabi, and learning from experiences and feedback from students, I have come to understand teaching as a process of careful disruptions.

I entered the academe not as a trained teacher but as a research activist, who was more used to speaking as an advocate than giving lectures. Almost without realising, I adopted a radical pedagogy with a strong notion of care and responsibility in the transmission of my activist knowledge and practice mixed with my interpretation of academic texts. I have written elsewhere how this caused a small storm in my institute when I was course leader of the institute's main MA course.[4] But over time, through writing and sharing my concerns about how to teach critical development studies, I found I was not alone. There are allies and co-conspirators, including within my institute, who see teaching as a way to provide hope and inspiration for collective transformation, rooted in pain and anger but fired by vision and dreams as part of critical development studies.

Before discussing the conundrums around development education, I first need to explain some key concepts which inform what I mean by teaching as a process of radical connection through careful disruptions. The boundaries between activism and academe are messy, especially in the classroom where what counts as knowledge and what is considered teachable is always contested. There is an element of vulnerability to sharing your passions and concerns in any space, but particularly when you are the convenor of that space as a teacher and 'expert' and especially as the big questions about economic, ecological and social injustice do not have easy answers. Such vulnerability is a radical way to connect with students. Activist scholar Richa Nagar describes how she mobilises radical vulnerability in her classroom to enable deep engagements and connections with students (Nagar et al. 2023). She invites her students to learn from grassroots theatre and storying to co-create and dream together. Radical vulnerability is a collective journey of unlearning and relearning where the teacher acts as facilitator and co-learner. As Nagar states, it is possible to transform 'the spaces of learning, unlearning and relearning by embracing radical vulnerability as a mode of being and growing together... Thus, radical vulnerability becomes an episteme – a way to feel, connect, and relate; a way to find trust, hope, and meaning; a way to dream, dismantle, and co-create in the big and small moments' (ibid., 267).

In today's neoliberal university the politics of the classroom also means challenging the university itself as a gendered, racialised and class-based institution founded in colonialism. Universities are today turning rapidly into privatised corporate-run knowledge production centres, where 'cultural values have been rephrased in economic rather than political terms' (Goodman 2021: 23).

To adopt radical vulnerability as a position when teaching in a European (Global North) development studies institute means to be willing to call out Eurocentrism and its erasure of other knowledges in academia and everyday life (Sundberg 2014: 34). It means being unafraid to point out the fissures in dominant development discourses and to encourage students to engage in encounters with diverse life-worlds and consider their co-responsibilities. In other words, to recognise different forms of knowledge as necessarily requiring action. It means being open to conversing with, walking alongside non-dominant epistemic worlds; 'moving, engaging, reflecting' on the plurality of knowledge (ibid., 59). As feminist ecologist Juanita Sundberg states, teaching means to leave 'one's comfortable psychological, political, and discursive place' (ibid., 70) in order to engage honestly with others discursively and politically.

This reframing of teaching as a practice formed by relational and accountable connections requires students and teachers to understand their own positionality. I have found Aimee Carillo Rowe's writing (2005, 2008) on differential belonging helpful in understanding the politics of teaching as a form of connection and building relations of trust. Carillo Rowe analyses the politics of relations across racial, gender, class and other boundaries within academia. As she states, in the classroom it is important to understand how,

> The sites of our belonging constitute how we see the world, what we value, who we are (becoming). The meaning of self is never individual, but a shifting set of relations that we move in and out of . . . My work aims to render transparent the political conditions and effects of our belonging, where we place our bodies, and with whom we build our affective ties. I call this placing a 'politics of relation'.
>
> Carillo Rowe 2005: 16

My positionality as a white older woman with dual Global North citizenship teaching students mostly from the Global South requires me to be aware of location and body/knowledge/status positioning. It means I must unlearn my sense of belonging to whiteness as entitlement. I also need to consider how age, gender and class converge in an embodied way through my role as a teacher who is in authority but who wishes to speak from a place of vulnerability, connection and care. Similarly, students mostly coming from the Global South are often learning to be racialised for the first time in the Dutch context, while still being part of an elite who are attending a Global North institution. They belong simultaneously to oppressed and privileged groups in fluid ways which are made more complex in conversations about embodied, racialised and gendered injustice as part of development studies. As Carillo Rowe states, the key to differential belonging is not to conflate identity and politics but to grapple with the different positionalities and relate those positions to larger social and political connections: 'Interrogating the politics of our belonging is something that anyone can do and all of us should do, regardless of the degree to which we are privileged' (ibid., 36). More dramatically, she states that 'embracing' differential belonging is 'a vehicle for healing by empowering us to cross the lines of separation that deaden and wound' (ibid., 38).

These insights by Nagar, Sundberg and Carillo Rowe underline how we need to unsettle dominant narratives of development and see development studies as a contested set of ideas and practices as we address historical silences and violences. Critical pedagogy that carefully disrupts development's material and discursive powers means challenging the 'deeply-rooted hierarchies, asymmetric power structures, the universalization of Western knowledge, the privileging of whiteness, and the taken-for-granted Othering of the majority world' (Sultana 2019: 33). Using pedagogies to disentangle 'hegemonic ideologies and representations, from colonialist logics and practices, and decentering of Eurocentric knowledges and ways of being' (ibid., 35) openly questions power and privileges, including those that circulate in the classroom. Feminist geographer Farhana Sultana describes this form of teaching as one of 'critical hope' where 'meaningful dialogue and empathic responses in the classroom foster possibilities of social justice, for environmental justice, for equitable relations, and more hope-full futures' (ibid.). Sultana sees the academy as a place of political action which can undercut 'a sense of despair and inaction when a problem is overwhelming in order to have impacts beyond the academy and into the future' (Sultana 2022: np). She is hopeful that development studies can tackle systemic racism, xenophobia and ecocide. Teaching can encourage 'powerful acts of solidarity and radical care that can inspire, reimagine, and co-create change' (ibid.).

Critical hope also underlies the pedagogies of several courses which I have co-taught. One such course, 'Transitions to Social Justice LAB', was designed to disrupt the prevailing academic 'business as usual' during lockdown in Covid-19. Now held in-person, the course fosters connections among students and the teaching staff through 'nurturing words and conversations, healing visual and poetic horizons' organised around actions of 'refusing, learning, eating, caring, healing, and nurturing' rather than traditional academic themes (Icaza and Sheik 2023: 205).

The course looks at the process of transition in the context of rising fundamentalisms, geopolitics, racism, sexism, homophobia, exclusions and marginalisations. From an embodied and place-based perspective, students are invited to consider the possibilities of 'an ethical life in a world that is deeply divided between those who consume and those who are consumed, including the life of others and the life of Earth'. [5] The classes are run as creative collective spaces of learning and unlearning, co-creating in the classroom a politics of knowledge of what the course leader sees as 'resistance studies'.

In my contribution to the course I facilitate two sessions on 'caring for the earth'. I invite students to 'reworld, reimagine, relive and reconnect with each other in order to care for the earth by fostering cross-cultural human and more than human well-being'. Our dialogues are inspired by Indigenous and ecofeminist thinkers and centre on the collective possibilities for rethinking life-in-common.[6] The sessions encourage a humble form of learning which looks at embodied and place-based connections of care with nature. Following a methodology proposed by the reading 'Manifestings', the aim of the session is to explore how people are connected to more-than-human beings in place, whether it is care for pets or house plants, river spirits or ancestral forests (Hernández et al. 2021: 858). The conversations lead to expressions of emotions about the loss of biodiversity and cultural knowledge, as well as affection for loved beings. There is also silence, nostalgia and wistfulness, along with anger about how so many beings are impacted by changes that disrupt relations of care. We discuss how it is possible to build relationships with more-than-human others and how, in spaces of vulnerability and reflection, it becomes possible to 'locate colonial-capitalist violence and its effects on ourselves and kin' (ibid., 859).

These descriptions of what I teach offer a sliver of the possibilities of connection, co-creation and relationship-building in the classroom. Other activist scholars have written about their teaching along the borders of academe and activism.[7] My friend and collaborator, ecofeminist Giovanna Di Chiro, has undertaken long-running projects that have engaged her students together with local communities in shared environmental activist projects (Barca et al. 2023). She teaches 'kin-centric environmental justice organising [as] an active, embodied approach for building critical connections' in tangible ways so that students learn directly 'interdependence and collective care'.[8] Di Chiro positions her teaching practice in the colonised places, geographies and community ecologies where she lives on the land of the Lenape (Pennsylvania, US). Di Chiro is inspired by Potawatomi botanist Robyn Wall Kimmerer (whom we discussed in Chapter 3). Kimmerer writes that we need to live as if we'll be here 'for the long haul' and 'to take care of the land as if our lives, both spiritual and material, depended on it' (Kimmerer 2013: 9). An example of Di Chiro's 'kin-centric relationships' is a campus-community collaborative called Serenity Soular, which brings solar technology, sustainable community development and solar jobs training opportunities to residents in North Philadelphia, a majority-Black section of the city (Di Chiro and Rigell 2018).[9] Another example is the work of her students over the years with Chester residents to shut down the largest waste incinerator in the country and transition towards a zero waste economy in the region.

The conundrum in undertaking this kind of teaching is that it requires energy and demanding ethical care work, which is rarely acknowledged in academe. It takes years of engagement to foster change, as well as the time and funds to allow students to participate in community activities, none of which are priorities of neoliberal universities. Universities are now run as businesses, students are perceived as clients or customers, academics as experts, the funding priority is for STEM subjects rather than humanities and social sciences. Instead of time and money to work on political projects aiming at transitions towards sustainable societies and economies, there are a growing number of administrators and training units within universities hired to ensure efficient performance of academics measured by research and grant metrics (Truscott and Khoo 2024). All of this undermines academic freedom and the critical thinking that is required for critical development studies (Kapoor 2023: 354).

However, there are still some spaces that foster critical development. From 2020 to 2024 I participated in an international European Cooperation in Science and Technology (COST Action) on 'Decolonising Development',[10] which brought together nearly 100 academics engaged in critical development studies in universities around Europe. I was involved in the working group on teaching, which looked at how development studies could be a critical intellectual space and a site of activism with political and social relevance.[11] The network's goal was to confront the colonial legacy of development studies and to bring in non-Western and subaltern/ Indigenous texts, writers and practices to more inclusive and interdisciplinary teaching practice. In exposing Eurocentric and 'white normativity' the network shared its experiences of epistemic and ontological struggles in the face of neoliberalisation and corporatisation of the university. We looked at collective strategies to confront racism and gender-based violence in the academe, and more broadly how to end socio-economic barriers to higher education, calling attention to the colonial histories underlying global events such as the war in Ethiopia, Sudan, Ukraine and Palestine. The network created spaces for memorable encounters. For example, in 2022 and 2023 I attended two summer schools which were opportunities to create a collective process of unlearning/relearning (Cancar 2023: np). We spent three days exploring different pedagogies and understandings of development processes across disciplines, sharing personal stories and mapping out our connections and divergences. Such encounters and connections that spin out from unconventional learning practices are precious.[12]

Critical development studies is more and more engaging in sustained collaborative action to reorient and change values based on different sets of world views, practices and policies, even as it moves to the margins of academic institutions. For example, activist scholars like Ashish Kothari, the founder of the transnational civil society network the 'global tapestry of alternatives',[13] bring to academic spaces such as the Cost Action Summer Schools[14] examples of grassroots, grounded, bottom-up and participatory visioning processes. The network's focus on 'solidarity and reciprocity, diversity, freedom and autonomy, respect and responsibility, living with nature' (Kothari 2024: np)[15] provides examples of how care for others operates in marginal spaces worldwide. The examples show how communities that recentre care are helping to decommodify health, education, water and sanitation. This process is 'recommoning life in general and care work in particular, challenging class and racial disparity, learning from communities' as well as building a 'deeper awareness of systemic social justice issues' (Cave 2024: 1).

Section Three: *Repositioning care*

In this third section, as a conclusion to the chapter and book, I reflect on how development discourse (including teaching) should connect more fruitfully to care in ways that would change development practice profoundly. As we have seen throughout the book, 'care is a slippery word' (Tronto 2017: 31). To care implies a set of actions, connections and relations. It is work, an emotion, a disposition, a declaration of love, a politics for social and ecological justice through solidarity and collective action and hopes for conviviality. As Joan Tronto states, we need 'to have the courage to return to a forestalled alternative future, one in which care truly matters' (Tronto 2017: 39). So, what does it mean to care in development practice? Is it possible to focus care in transformative social and ecological just pathways towards sustainable development?

In pointing to practices of care I have been cautious in the book not to romanticise care as an innocent and self-evidently desirable set of values, but have tried to show the conundrums of how care refers to different meanings and practices. Each chapter took up a different set of meanings around care. In Chapter 2 we looked at care work making visible who does the work of caring, for whom and in which context as feminist economists revalue care. In Chapter 3 we explored the more-than-human relations of Earthcare, learning from ecofeminists, feminist political ecologists and critical Indigenous scholars about care meaning far more than naturalised assumptions about women caring for vulnerable people or the planet. In Chapter 4 we engaged in dialogues about care for future generations, asking whether it matters how many people are on this planet, looking at planetary boundaries and choices around bearing children. In Chapter 5 we explored interspecies care, looking at reciprocity in the interactions between humans and more-than-humans, including soil's relations with biodiversity and how humans can build qualitatively different relationships with the rest of the living world. In Chapter 6 we looked at how to learn about collective care from community economies, feminist, queer and ecological activist practices. We explored communally caring practices, based on 'well-being, safety through solidarity, trust and friendship, vulnerability and consent, tenderness, reciprocity, accessibility, kindness' (Ojeda et al. 2022: 13).

What we see in these diverse meanings and practices of care is that care is above all political. There is the promise of care to revolutionise how we live together in this world if people were to take up collective caring responsibilities that end inequalities of race, gender, age and ethnicity. Seeing care as political means being attentive to power relations and to the profound conundrum that care is part of our traditional structures 'while simultaneously already embodying the alternatives we fight and yearn for' (Anarcha Feminism 2022: 10–11).[16] We have to find trust, solidarity and reciprocity in caring relationships grounded in 'everyday making of relationships and relationalities' while also 'acknowledging the structural power inequalities underpinning care' (Tronto 2013: np). The politics of care means 'dealing with unavoidable tensions and conflicts' (Ojeda et al. 2022: 12). And it means moving beyond the nation state because 'as long as the nation state remains the container within which care is allocated then global unjust inequalities of care will exist' (Tronto 2013: np).

As we ponder what care means for development, particularly in today's ominous geo-political shifts and changes, the conclusion to the book is that caring about, giving/receiving care and developing ethics and networks of care necessitate working through dilemmas and contradictions. In short, conundrums. We live on a planet made up of many worlds and development processes, and development teaching needs to find ways to reorientate our way of thinking about how western modernity is entangled in those many other worlds if we are to foster relationality and care for humans and more-than-human beings.

As Columbian/US scholar Arturo Escobar states:

Living relationally attuned to being (part of) Earth – seems to be an idea whose time has come ... revisiting the human from a perspective of care, is of foremost importance ... We find many expressions of this idea in feminist, environmental, and ethic movements *caring for the web of life*, in all its dimensions: the care, healing, and repairing of the bodies, territories, landscapes, communities, cities, and institutions that we all are and inhabit.

Escobar 2023: np[17]

In the book I have pointed to many such stories that speak of care as power, as healing, as relationality, as weaving collective knowledge, as teaching with care, in the move towards 'more just and ecologically sustainable futures' (Terry et al. 2023). As Guam activist Julian Aguon states, we need to build a new world rooted in reciprocity and mutual respect for the Earth and for one another,[18] In a world organised around 'care-with' or *homines curans* 'one in which care truly matters' (Tronto 2017: 39), care is relational, context-dependent and 'can be practiced in everyday spaces and heal colonial wounds everywhere' (ibid.).

If we are to bring care to development processes, one of the major conundrums is how non-Indigenous peoples can connect with care as they recognise the colonial wounds felt by Indigenous peoples. To connect with care, humbleness and respect with Indigenous peoples' knowledge and practices is necessary but difficult. As the many examples given in the book attest, listening to Indigenous peoples would mean changing dominant, universalising, extractive development processes. It would mean learning how nature is conceived, perceived and lived in non-western cultural and territory-based cosmogonies and contexts. It would change how we teach development studies as we take into account the past, present and future learning from different cosmologies. Such alternative knowledges could shift what decolonial scholar Catherine Walsh describes as 'western modernity's universalized project of anthropocentric, masculine-centric, and secular separation, independence, and no-relation' (Walsh 2022: 137).

Learning offers inspiration for deep transformation because it is centred on care. Navajo sculptor, painter, printmaker and professor Melanie Yazzie describes Indigenous traditions as 'a radical power of kinship to inspire our dreams of liberation, the desire to build a world structured by relations of care, love, and abundance instead of relations of abandonment, harm, and scarcity' (Yazzie 2023: 601). She argues that 'caretaking must be at the centre of our collective efforts to build a future on a planet that is on the precipice of ruin. We must develop caretaking economies, caretaking ecologies, and caretaking geographies to restore the health of our land and water relatives and, ultimately, stand for life' (ibid., 603). She points to the 'countless ... Black, Indigenous, trans, migrant, and refugee freedom fighters' (ibid.) that are intricately involved in this radical care work.

Such stories of resistance and care counter mainstream universalising narratives of development as linear growth and progress. It is possible to expose how colonialism, racism and classism underline development processes as 'scientists, technology developers, and environmental and social policymakers support alternately extracting or "stewarding" natural and human resources' (Tall Bear 2019: 36). Sisseton Wahpeton Oyate professor Kim Tall Bear proposes 'making kin as an alternative approach to liberal multiculturalism, for righting relations gone bad.

If you/we are to live together in a good way here – as kin or as Peoples in alliance with reciprocal responsibilities to one another and to our other-than-human relatives with whose land, water, and animal bodies we are co-constituted' (ibid.).

I will now return to Deborah Bird Rose, whose work has so inspired me in my exploration of the conundrums of care. Her last book, published posthumously, is a study of Indigenous philosophy examined through an ecological lens, where ecology is understood as the connectivities of different beings in a living world. Her work helps us to understand how to learn from Indigenous relations which are 'predicated on care and the mutual connectivity of all life' (Jolly 2024: 33), and which '[unite] human and non-human, body and spirit, ideal and real' (ibid., 25). As Bird Rose describes it:

> To be seriously alive, then, is to be in connection. Not only does the person, or organism, or Country, live from one moment to the next; they also contribute to the lives of others and gain benefit from the lives of others. To be seriously alive is to be complexly connected in relationships that sustain systems of life.
>
> Bird Rose 2024: 49

Care and solidarity are integral to remaking, resistance, re-envisioning and learning from grounded experiences and lived realities of communities globally. Another conundrum is that paying attention to complex holistic connections means there are no straightforward pathways. Our knowledge of relations and connection is necessarily determined by context, space and history and therefore the connections are always partial and changing. Development needs to find ways to recognise the interconnections among living things in the practices that build pathways for transformation open to diverse imaginaries and practices 'flourishing in the cracks and fissures of oppressive designs and practices linked to colonial capitalism and extraction' (Escobar 2023: np).

Such imaginaries work against the development mainstream vision 'building rhizomes in multiple directions with like-minded experiments, concepts and struggles . . . creating pluriversal kinds of collective intelligence on the heels of digitality; meditating on and organizing horizontally for the phasing out of a civilization premised on bioeconomic narratives and capitalist hegemony' (ibid.).

As I have shown in this book, I have come across a myriad of ways people are making caring connections with all living things. Such careful connections enable us to go through the storms we are facing and the ones development studies and development teaching, in practice and theory, need to confront.

Conundrums of connecting with care

Caring to maintain, continue and repair our world means connecting with others and extending our sense of self to be part of collective thinking that envisions new possibilities. Writing this book I have been acutely aware of how difficult this is as facts and data blur and mix with emotions, memories and intentions of different kinds. I wrote as the Ukraine War erupted, as we witnessed the horrific Hamas attacks on 7 October 2023 and appalling genocide of Palestinian people, and as the war spread to other places in the Middle East, extreme levels of violence in places like Sudan, Yemen, Ethiopia, Myanmar and Mexico, along with a shoring up of authoritarian regimes as right-wing parties won Europe, including the places I live in Italy and the Netherlands. And in November 2024 Trump won a resounding Republican trifecta and is destroying hard-won rights and fatally disrupting geo-political relations.

Living in the Global North I felt how hard it was to shake off post-pandemic loneliness as many continue to retreat into online worlds. Even in the wealthy Global North where I live, economic, social and material uncertainty is rising for young people and those facing marginalisation of old age. The climate crisis has seen an increase in global floods, fires, extreme heat and unrelenting loss of biodiversity. But as US feminist and journalist Rebecca Solnit (2024) states, it is possible to be heartbroken and hopeful. People do care about the loss of human life and culture, of forests, of plants, animals, lakes. Behind the care is anger, which can drive us to resist. Solnit invites us to 'lay up our supplies of love, care, trust community and resolve' (2024: np). She also points to the need for stillness and quiet times to recharge, and to find community to build strength through relationships with people we trust. During my life I have learnt from the environment and women's movements of the 1980s, the anti-globalisation movements of the 1990s, the Indigenous leadership in the climate movements of the 2000s and have seen in the last decade how feminist, queer, trans and anti-racist movements have profoundly changed conversations.

In a world of turmoil with the rise of far-right, anti-gender, anti-'immigrant' politics reeling from the impact of wars, genocides, climate change and now Trumpian shocks, new kinds of knowledge and new kinds of conversations are needed that resist, bear witness and walk in allyship together. Solidarity built from a plurality of voices can strengthen communities of care, reimagine futures and create new worlds that resist and counter destructive forces. New thinking needs to build on hope arising from diverse experiences and theoretical openness while remaining aware of intersectional differences of environments, class, gender, race and sexuality rooted in histories of colonialism.

Such stories of hope and resistance are and can continue to be woven, lived and taught. We need to take heart from those that inspire. I have been humbled by many. Listening to them I have felt emboldened to speak from my own context, history and time, with an embodied voice entangled with so many other lives. I have aimed to provide a guide to stories that inspire, to point to the conundrums of care, woven through the shared histories and knowledges, from so many diverse places. My aim has been to be brief, not heavily theory laden, but accessible and engaging – sharing my own personal reflections – so that readers will want to continue to dive into the debates and into their own lived connections and conundrums of care.

Epilogue

When I was completing this book, I met with a former colleague in Rome during that period of recovery between Christmas and New Year, where you walk off rich meals, escape the emotions of family closeting and endure the bewildering sense that you have lost a hold on time, or at least what day of the week it is. We strolled along the cobblestones of Monti, the area where we had worked together in an international NGO nearly three decades ago. We were reminiscing, regretting the encroachment of tourism while still enjoying the beauty of ancient buildings silhouetted against sweeping blue December skies. We fell immediately into puzzling about how could it have happened? We had understood the dangers of globalisation for the environment, for people, for the planet in the 1990s. Yet, we had dismally failed to avert it. At the INGO we had led research projects, wrote articles, lobbied in UN and other global venues for alternatives to top-down, Northern-centric unsustainable development. We recalled for the nth time the dramatic moment in May 1997 at the final plenary of our organization's 22nd World Conference in Santiago di Compostela so hopefully entitled 'Which globalisation? Opening spaces for civic engagement'.[1] The audience of many hundreds had gathered to listen to an array of distinguished speakers, including five leaders of UN agencies. We recalled how we had clutched each other, close to tears, as we watched the heads of the UN defeat the keynote speakers we had invited. They tore apart the speakers' plea for a freeing of imagination and for marginal voices to be brought to the centre of development debates. The UN heads scoffed at the capabilities of poor and local political processes to shape globalisation. They rebutted any elegant arguments about culture and justice led by the Global South. Experts, they argued, were needed to design effective economic and political institutions. Local communities did not understand how power operated.

When we had set up the debate, we had thought our keynotes would easily convince leaders of the UN agencies and Bretton Woods institutions that many worlds could exist together, and that a more equitable and democratic vision was needed to replace the failure of the global development project. We had hoped that the Conference would build bridges that could forge new imaginations, new alliances that would impact the 'real world' as old politics would be reshaped into a new multifarious politics beyond parties and beyond multilateral institutions.

No doubt we were naïve, not strategic nor powerful enough, but as Cora Coralina[2] stated: 'Even when everything seems to fall apart, it is up to us to decide whether to laugh or cry, go or stay, give up or fight; because we discover, along with life's uncertain path, that the most important thing is to decide.'[3]

My colleague and I decided to continue, in other venues, in other ways. He is currently working with large companies in Europe in the arena of corporate responsibility pushing for a sustainable green transition. In my teaching, transnational and local activism I chose to continue to fight for gender equity and environmental justice and hope for change.

This book is a testament to my belief that it is possible to interweave words and actions to resist and survive and to honour the promise of life's continuity. Throughout the book I share how I have been influenced by many brilliant thinkers, places and beings. Each chapter starts with a quote that inspired me, and I refer in the text and in endnotes to the people who have guided me, some whom I have known personally, others whom I have read or whom I have encountered online. Their collective wisdom enables me to care, as part of my feminist politics and personal survival. As I was researching for the book, I read an article that reminded me how I have written elsewhere that social and environmental resilience is possible when guided by the principles of care. While kindly ascribing the thought to me, the authors wrote more astutely than I did, 'when coupled with the politics and practices of care, resilience can be rethought as a feminist transformative device' (Gregoratti et al. 2024, 1).

Resilience is a difficult word. While we can remain hopeful about life's continuity, we are facing huge challenges. Samantha Harvey in her extraordinary book *Orbital*, which won the Man Booker Prize in 2024, puts it starkly: 'The planet is shaped by the sheer amazing force of human want, which has changed everything, the forests, the poles, the reservoirs, the glaciers, the rivers, the seas, the mountains, the coastlines, the skies, a planet contoured and landscaped by want' (Harvey 2024).

How do we counter this huge want and greed of the forces of production (rather than reproduction)?

My slim book is a modest offering to a collective countering of these forces. I highlight a few of the continued efforts of resistance and resilience in the politics and practice of care in feminist and other allies' work. As I was revising the book I was engaged in conversations, workshops, on and offline that built on the fertile imagination of feminists around the world. These included: online conversations with members of the Duke University project on 'Revaluing Care in the Global Economy'[4] that brings together gender studies, feminist economics, art and sexuality into research on care; discussions on feminist care and resistance in the neoliberal university with my friends at the Decolonizing Development Cost Action; a conversation with members of the Minerva Lab based in Rome on feminist methodologies; a hybrid launch in Delft of a methodologically daring feminist *Handbook on gender and water* in Delft; and an online launch of a new network on Feminist Agroecology connecting Indian women farmers and European feminist political ecologists.

These encounters make me realise that writing a book is only ever a beginning when engaging in the politics of care. The book is embedded in an ongoing process of feminist transformative processes. I am grateful that possible contributions of the book are made easier by being freely available online due to the Erasmus University Rotterdam library open access programme. I plan to communicate further the collective insights of the book's chapters via podcasts and blogs on websites.[5] I also plan to take the discussion into European and UN based policy and activist workshops, and to reach out to the various academic networks and transnational feminist meshworks that flow in and out of my life. My hope is that by using multiple channels the book will help to shape connections of care and flourishing for a better world.

Notes

Chapter 1: Caring Conversations: An Introduction

1 See https://www.juliet-artmagazine.com/en/the-hybrid-universe-of-patricia-piccinini/
2 WIDE is now called WIDE+ and while its focus has shifted towards issues around migration, it continues to promote inclusive and intersectional feminist movement building in Europe, in solidarity with feminists in the Global South. See https://wideplus.org/
3 The Wellbeing Ecology Gender cOmmunity (WEGO) innovative training network funded by the European Union's Horizon 2020 research and innovation programme under the Marie Sklodowska-Curie grant agreement No. 764908-WEGO 2018-2021. In the book I refer to several of the participants' writings and the collective writings we did together. For more information see https://www.wegoitn.org/
4 I use Global North and Global South referring not so much to geography but rather to the dominance of geopolitical powers – these are more usual terms used in development discourse than minority and majority world.
5 See Elizabeth DeLoughrey's (2021) sweeping article on 'the long and deep history of feminist theories of care' in the disciplines of 'ethics, politics, ontology, ecology, psychology, race, sexuality, labor, and maternity' (812). See also the interesting discussion of resilience and care in recent debates on feminist theory (Gregoratti et al., 2024), including reference to my own argument that care can overhaul the inequalities resulting from resource extractivism, potentially leading to fairer, more resilient and more sustainable lives.
6 I have learnt from conversations over the years with my decolonial colleagues Rosalba Icaza and Agustina Solera about the importance of being open to otherwise ways of knowing.

Chapter 2: Care Work: Valuing Social Reproduction

1. I met Elke Krasny just as she had finished writing the book and we have since enjoyed several exchanges across our different academic fields in The Hague and in Vienna. She is a Professor at the Academy of Fine Arts, Vienna as well as a curator, cultural theorist and urban researcher.
2. The essay by Arundhati Roy, 'The pandemic is a portal', 3 April 2020 – see https://www.ft.com/content/10d8f5e8-74eb-11ea-95fe-fcd274e920ca – was an inspiration for many.
3. See the Duke University project website on 'revaluing care' led by Jocelyn Olcott: https://www.revaluingcare.org/
4. Based on conversations held in 2021 and 2022, the names have been anonymised.
5. Filipinos are the most in demand domestic workers in Italy, valued in a stereotypical way of hard-working Asians, speaking English, as religious and polite. Many come on government schemes to Italy, and are provided training in the Philippines before they leave and are registered with the Filipino Embassy in Rome (Collantes 2016).
6. See the Italian Statistics Bureau ISTAT figures: https://noi-italia.istat.it/
7. The 2011 film called *Cose Dell'Altro Mondo* (Out of this World) – a mainstream comedy by Francesco Patierno – depicted the impact on the northern Italian city of Treviso if all the migrants were to disappear overnight. There were scenes (both bewildering and funny) of grey-haired older people in various states of disarray wandering the city streets lost without their migrant carers, and their Italian families at their wit's ends as to what to do.
8. This section is based on a joint paper which we gave at the International Association of Feminist Economics in Rome in June 2024, based on the MA student's activist research on care organisations.
9. I was introduced to Manuela Zechner's work by colleagues of the WEGO-ITN network who work with her closely.
10. Zechner writes as an activist, journalist and researcher; see: https://roarmag.org/essays/barcelona-en-comu-guanyem/; https://radicalcollectivecare.blogspot.com/2015/03/about-radical-collective-

care-practices.html; https://heteropolitics.net/wp-content/uploads/2020/12/Case-Studies-in-Spain.pdf
11 Zechner describes the term 'Cuidadania' coined by Spanish feminist movements to re-frame citizenship ('ciudadania') as a matter of care ('cuidado') – also seen in the vignette from Chile.
12 These proposals I selected from various feminist statements about the impact of Covid-19 – I looked for those that focused on care and raised economic as well as ecological concerns. Krasny in her book labels these manifestos as part of 'care feminism' (Krazny 2022).
13 See: https://humanservices.hawaii.gov/wp-content/uploads/2020/04/4.13.20-Final-Cover-D2-Feminist-Economic-Recovery-D1.pdf
14 See: https://warwick.ac.uk/fac/soc/law/research/centres/globe/policybriefs/pb7_towards_feminist_recovery_plans_for_covid19_and_beyond_-_serena_natile_feb22.pdf
15 See: https://www.unwomen.org/en/digital-library/publications/2021/09/beyond-covid-19-a-feminist-plan-for-sustainability-and-social-justice
16 There are several academic reviews of responses to Covid-19 by care feminism. See *Signs*, *Feminist Studies* or *Feminist Economics*, which produced special issues on the pandemic. Michael Fine and Joan Tronto guest edited a special issue of the *International Journal of Care and Caring*, published in 2022, entitled 'Care, caring, and the global Covid-19 pandemic'.

Chapter 3: Earthcare: Ecofeminist and Indigenous Approaches to Our Life-worlds

1 See the website of WEDO https://wedo.org/ which details the advocacy work of the organisation in the spirit of Bella Abzug.
2 The Right Livelihood Award is an international award to 'honour and support those offering practical and exemplary answers to the most urgent challenges facing us today'. https://rightlivelihood.org/ Maathai won the Award in 1984 and Shiva in 1993.
3 See Vandana Singh's powerful recollection of the Chipko Movement and its resistance to loggers throughout the Himalayas in the 1970s.

She describes its 'rallying cry for collective self-determination and environmental protection' as larger and more profound than individualist western conceptions of nature (Singh 2021: xix).
4 Irene Leonardelli successfully defended her PhD in 2023 and is now doing her post-doctoral research.
5 See the website: https://www.theoceanandus.org
6 Plumwood Inc. continues the legacy of Val Plumwood through a not-for-profit trust organisation which hosts writers' retreats that continue her work to challenge human exceptionalism and to build ecological communities. Recently Plumwood Mountain was officially transferred to the Batemans Bay Local Aboriginal Land Council and Walbunja custodianship. See: https://www.abc.net.au/news/2024-09-24/val-plumwood-estate-handed-back-to-walbunja-traditional-owners/104384170
7 See also the article on the 'speculative turn' in anthropology and the (re)colonisation of indigeneity (Chandler and Reid 2020).
8 See for example the video on songspirals: https://bawakacollective.com/audio-visual-songspirals/
9 I was introduced to Kimmerer's work by members of the WEGO network and have used her work since in my teaching, and like many others am deeply inspired by her writing. See: https://www.robinwallkimmerer.com/
10 See the Intercontinental Cry media platform: https://intercontinentalcry.org/ and Miriam Lang's (2022) study on Buen Vivir as a territorial practice. Building a more just and sustainable life through interculturality in the Cayambe looks at relations between human and nonhuman life, and care for the local ecosystems, especially for soil fertility and water sources.

Chapter 4: Caring about Having Babies: Reproductive Rights and Population Ethics

1 See the *Economist*, 22 July 2023.
2 See SisterSong, the largest national multi-ethnic Reproductive Justice collective, at https://www.sistersong.net/reproductive-justice

3 In the 1990s and 2000s I encountered many examples of population control programmes as I was writing and advocating for women's reproductive rights and choices in projects I was involved in with funding from UNFPA and other UN agencies. Some of these experiences I wrote about in a monograph on body politics (Harcourt 2009).

Chapter 5: Interspecies Care: Learning with the More-than-Human

1 I see queer ecology as helping to reshape our thinking about the connections among ecology, bodies and territories through its critique of the heteronormativity of science and subversion of mainstream environmentalism in its research around gender, race, sexuality and the human in relation to climate change, colonial capitalism and environmental toxicity.
2 In her 2017 preface Maria Puig de la Bellacasa states how she is influenced and has worked closely with other feminist scholars such as Donna Haraway and Anna Tsing.
3 There are other lively examples of feminists engaging with care for the soil both in practice and metaphorically. Jennifer Mae Hamilton and Astrida Neimanas (2018) play on the idea of composting between environmental humanities and feminism looking at the 'friability of contemporary environmental humanities soil in particular ways' (Hamilton and Neimanas 2018: 501). Neimanas later wrote with Laura McLauchlan about their experiences of teaching climate change in the classroom as a feminist issue, looking at the method of 'composting' from intersectional, anticolonial, queer and crip perspectives (Neimanas and McLauchlan 2022). Another study by Turner et al. 2024 looks at the emergence of a 'composting ethic' in Australia with community efforts to 'revitalise and grow city soils and advance anti-colonial food waste management through community composting' (Turner et al. 2024: 1). They see soil as underpinning 'human and planetary health and wellbeing' (ibid.). See also Krzywoszynska and Marchesi (2020) on the needs of soils.

4 For more on this and other citizen science projects on soils, see: https://oursoil.wp.rpi.edu/home/nuestrossuelos/
5 For example, Shruti Desai and Harriet Smith (2018) write about interspecies care in urban London. Their research investigates how people are learning to care for other species in games and experiences that promote ethical encounters with trees and animals. In an experiment with 'multispecies co-breathing' children learn to 'appreciate animals as both other-than-human and subject' and to enjoy an 'ethical encounter in being-with' the animals (Desai and Smith: 52). See also Pitt (2018), who discusses diverse relationships with more-than-humans in community gardening, arguing that there are diverse qualities of relating.
6 Based on discussions at the Rachel Carson Center's Multispecies Reading Group led by Thom van Dooren and Ursula Münster in 2015 and 2016.
7 Van Dooren co-wrote with Deborah Bird-Rose. For more on his extensive writing on human entanglements with threatened species and places, including crows living in other parts of the world, see his website: https://www.thomvandooren.org/
8 Crip theory brings together queer and disability studies, questioning systems of compulsory able-bodiedness and compulsory heterosexuality (McRuher 2006). I was introduced to crip theory by Ilenia Iengo, who used it in her PhD as part of the WEGO project.
9 https://www.sinsinvalid.org/mission
10 Similar approaches can be found in apocalyptic ecology; see https://www.apocalypticecology.com/
11 Peppa Pig is an animated character described as an anthropomorphic female piglet, who first appeared in 2004 on British TV and is now broadcast in 180 countries. Her You Tube channel has 38.1 million subscribers. See: https://www.youtube.com/channel/UCAOtE1V7Ots4DjM8JLlrYgg.
12 Black environmentalist from Lowndes County Alabama, Catherine Coleman Flowers, is an example of a woman activist fighting against racialised environmental neglect and injustice. Her book *Waste: One woman's fight against America's dirty secret* (2020) calls attention to how sewage and wastewater are connected to rural poverty, infrastructural

inequity and systemic racism in the neglected areas of rural southern USA.
13 Art is something I keep coming back to not as an artist, but as someone who is moved by art. I experimented with using art as part of feminist methodologies in a chapter I co-wrote and co-drew with a MA student; see Harcourt and Arguello Calle (2022).
14 For example, Pratt discusses Jeremijenko's Cross(x)Species Adventure Club, which is an art supper club that aims to explore human's gastronomical, economic and material interdependency with butterflies, worms, geese, bats and other intelligent and delicious creatures. See http://www.carbonarts.org/projects/crossx-species-adventure-club-australian-safari/
15 See the artist explain the project at https://www.miriamsimun.xyz/talks
16 See her 2011 TED Talk, viewed by nearly 2 million people by September 2024: https://www.ted.com/talks/jae_rhim_lee_my_mushroom_burial_suit?subtitle=en
17 For more about the Infinity Burial Suit by Coeio – a biodegradable burial shroud made from mushroom spores – see a blog post by Eirene Cremations: https://eirenecremations.com/blog/how-mushroom-burial-suit-works?srsltid=AfmBOorKNJyEplX8y7xPKUEqIaGNyE7wLlKPJSNFnCHltZlu1MnLlTOC

Chapter 6: Caring Communities: Building Reciprocity through Degrowth, Community Economies and Radical Care

1 Another example would have been citizen scientists concerned with environmental degradation working with communities to collect data on pollution – I decided not to include this group because the connection between data collection, the integrity of the results and the politics of what you do with the data is still a largely academic discussion (Hecker and Taddicken 2022).
2 Bue Rübner Hansen and Manuela Zechner (2020) point out how such meshworks are tied together through digital global practices. As well as

presenting an insightful analysis into how social media is embedded in our everyday life. They raise the concern about the environmental and ecological impact of the technical infrastructures of social media, which I do not address. See their article: 'Careless networks' in https://spheresjournal.org/wp-content/uploads/spheres-6_RuebnerHansen_Zechner.pdf

3 See: https://degrowth.info/en/conference/the-hague-2021
4 Julie Graham and Katherine Gibson have published together since their PhD days under the *nom de plume* of J. K. Gibson-Graham. I met them in 2004 at the Women and Politics of Place project referred to in Section One of this chapter. I have learnt much from the network since its founding in the 1990s. As a member of CERN I have attended some meetings in Italy, the Netherlands, Australia, Japan and the UK. CERN members held summer schools at the *Convento* in Bolsena (see Chapter 1) over several years before Covid-19 hit.
5 See the information on the 'Diverse Economies and Livable Worlds' book series: https://www.upress.umn.edu/search-grid/?series=diverse-economies-and-livable-worlds
6 See: https://www.communityeconomies.org
7 See the review of the community economies work on care in Dombroski, Healy and McKinnon 2018.
8 See the website: https://www.communityeconomies.org/take-back-economy
9 See also the *Commons Manifesto* Bauwens et al. (2019) and the classic critique of the commons by Massimo De Angelis (2017) and Silvia Federici and Georgis Caffentzis (2014).
10 All the quotations in this section come from the article dated 8 September 2022 by Zechner, which is an online magazine – *Berliner Gazette* – and does not have any page references. See https://after-extractivism.berlinergazette.de
11 See https://viacampesina.org/en/publication-the-path-of-peasant-and-popular-feminism-in-la-via-campesina/ See: https://viacampesina.org/en/25n23-with-conviction-we-pave-the-way-for-peasant-and-popular-feminism-build-food-sovereignty-and-fight-against-crises-and-violence/
12 See https://wiyiyaniuthangani.humanrights.gov.au/

13 See https://globalwomenstrike.net/
14 See the 2023 article by Kristina García on the archive at the University of Pennsylvania, which records the work of the Wages for Housework movement: https://penntoday.upenn.edu/news/true-value-womens-work-wages-for-housework#:~:text=The%20Wages%20for%20Housework%20movement,and%20carries%20on%20the%20work.
15 See: https://www.justtransitioncare.com/.
16 In 2011 I met Chloe Schwenke, who was a senior advisor at USAID during the Obama Administration and a member of the US Chapter of the Society for International Development. She shared with me her experiences as a transwoman and the difficulties she faced, the loneliness and the importance of community. I learnt a lot from her as we continued to correspond for a few years over how to recognise trans issues in gender and development. See her memoirs – *Self-ish: A Transgender Awakening* (2018).
17 See Elke Krasny and Helena Reckett, 'On Caring', New Alphabet School #4 Caring, 12 June 2020, https://www.hkw.de/en/app/mediathek/video/79091
18 I bring Murphy into the discussion here recalling a heated debate we had about care in the WEGO project during one of our training labs. Murphy's arguments were evoked when the idea of promoting care as a powerful feminist political process and also as a principled practice within the WEGO community was challenged as romantic, soft and maternalising.
19 I was visiting Katherine Gibson when revising the MS of this book and she kindly shared a draft of her and Kelly Dombroski's responses to the Handbook entitled 'Responding with and for joy', which is being featured in a forthcoming special issue of *Rethinking Marxism*.

Chapter 7: Connecting with Care: Pedagogies for Transformation

1 Being caring in my pedagogical approaches, opening my room to students and meeting them outside of the classroom and the institute is something

to which I can devote time as an established professor. As one of my younger colleagues pointed out, time to care is not part of the quantifiable incentives determining life for those on tenure track trajectories.

2   Serendipitously as I was writing this sentence, I received an unexpected email message from a male student in Ghana whom I had supervised some years back. He wrote about his job as an extension worker with women farmers and that he was 'grateful for the knowledge and understanding on the complexities of gender issue you impacted on me and now a tool in handling my day-to-day mandate'. Private Email correspondence 21 November 2024.

3   Taken from https://www.instagram.com/missenvyperu/p/C9fSYOXSAjQ/?img_index=1 16 July.

4   See Harcourt 2017 and the exchange that followed between myself and an ISS PhD student in the *Third World Quarterly*, where I had to reflect further on the course and my pedagogical position (Harcourt 2018).

5   From the course outline by my colleague Rosalba Icaza for the course taught from 2022 to 2023.

6   The texts are 'Caring as Country' (Suchet-Pearson et al. 2013) and 'The Creatures Collective: Manifestings' (Hernández et al. 2021), together with the video: https://bawakacollective.com/audio-visual-songspirals/ The readings and video invite reflection on connection to Earthothers and how it is possible to re-envision how to reworld, reimagine, relive and reconnect with each other in order to care for the Earth.

7   For example, Bethaney Turner shared her work with students on community gardens at the Liviana Conference 2024. See Turner et al. 2024.

8   Taken from my notes from a talk Di Chiro gave at the ISS in June 2024. See also her 2006 article on teaching urban ecology, where she addresses the dilemmas of a socially decontextualised nature by taking students into nearby toxic environments to collect data on the local community's health; the data collected by the students was shared with the community.

9   https://generocity.org/philly/2018/03/07/serenity-soular-north-philadelphia-solar-states-swarthmore-college/

10 Cost Action is a European Union fund that supports interdisciplinary research networks for four years to investigate a theme in an 'Action'. See

https://www.cost.eu/about/about-cost/ The focus of the 'Action' I joined was decolonising development, which was defined as 'the challenge to reconstruct development . . . a resetting and diversification of the structures, institutions and spaces in which knowledge about and for development is produced, shared, contested and put into practice': https://decolonise.eu/about-us-cost-action-decolonising-development/
11 See the Cost Action 'Decolonising development' statement of shared values: https://decolonise.eu/understanding-of-shared-values/
12 See another example of unconventional teaching practices from Zechner, *The Future Archive*, at https://thisappearance.wordpress.com/2014/11/02/the- future-archive/ And also the course channeling the book *Forces of reproduction* by Stefania Barca: https://www.youtube.com/playlist?list=PLvSbE4v4CV7fJ_jmaPHWsjsd1it5nEVsb
13 See: https://globaltapestryofalternatives.org/
14 I knew Smitu Kothari, Ashish Kothari's older brother, very well in my earlier career. It was such a pleasure to meet Ashish in the last few years in conferences on degrowth and political ecology as well as at the Summer Schools in Kassel, and once briefly in Pune. We found we shared political connections as well as vivid memories of his brother, who worked tirelessly for tribal peoples.
15 He describes the work of Vikalp Sangam (VP), a national network/platform in India which documents collaborations amongst ninety grassroots groups involved in creating alternative frameworks for justice, equity and ecological sustainability. Their meetings, or Sangams, are safe spaces including no tolerance for sexual or other forms of harassment or discrimination (ibid). VP is linked to the broader platform: Global Tapestry of Alternatives, a project founded by Kothari with others, and focuses on bringing together local and regional networks of radical alternatives.
16 See Nicole Rose: https://rootsandall.co.uk/podcast/episode-57-nicole-rose-of-solidarity-apothecary/ who uses plant medicines to 'strengthen collective autonomy, self-defence and resilience to climate change, capitalism and state violence' (https://solidarityapothecary.org/). Care as a radical act can be seen in ecofeminist manifestos such as the 'Manifesto on Economies of Care' by Navdanya, the organisation founded by

Vandana Shiva. The Navdanya Manifesto refers to 'Earth Care' in terms of all life forms being in relation with each other. Economies of care means that local economies are where 'sustenance, health and wellbeing converge and regenerate' in ways that create 'harmony and prosperity'. See https://navdanyainternational.org/wp-content/uploads/2023/11/Manifesto-Making-Peace-with-the-Earth-DWD-Rev5.pdf

17 I have enjoyed a warm friendship with Arturo Escobar since we met, now over thirty years ago in 1993. We wrote together in the 1990s and 2000s and he encouraged me to enter academia as a second career in my fifties. It was only when I joined the university that I realised what an influence he was in critical development studies, and beyond.

18 Julian Aguon's book *No country for eight-spot butterflies* (2022) tells his and the peoples of the Pacific's stories of resistance and resilience in the age of climate disaster. See: https://www.julianaguon.com For more on the ongoing colonial struggles in Guam see: https://www.theguardian.com/world/2020/aug/08/our-childrens-lives-on-the-line-the-ongoing-battle-for-guam

Epilogue

1 The conference speeches and reflections can be found in the journal *Development* 4 (4) (December 1997) 'Globalization: Responses from Santiago'.

2 A Brazilian poet and writer who became famous in her seventies and continues to be a feminist icon for Brazilian women and girls.

3 This wonderful quote was shared with me as a New Year greetings for 2025 by CEPIA, a local human rights NGO in Brazil, the founder of which has been a friend since the early 1990s. See their website: https://cepia.org.br/

4 See https://www.revaluingcare.org/

5 Many of the websites have been mentioned in the book, for example: the WEGO website, Undisciplined Environments, Community Economies Research Network, Degrowth.info.

References

1 Caring conversations: An Introduction

DeLoughrey, E. (2021), 'Care', *Women's Studies*, 50 (8): 812–819, DOI: 10.1080/00497878.2021.1994317

Fernandes, S. (2017), *Curated stories: the uses and misuses of storytelling*, New York: Oxford University Press.

Gregoratti, C., M. Linnell and M.A. Caretta (2024), 'Resilience: why should we think with care?', *Global Social Challenges Journal* (early view): 1–9, DOI: 10.1332/27523349Y2024D000000033

Haraway, D. (2011), 'Speculative fabulations for technoculture's generations: Taking care of unexpected country', *Australian Humanities Review*. Available online: https://australianhumanitiesreview.org/2011/05/01/speculative-fabulations-for-technocultures-generations-taking-care-of-unexpected-country/ (Accessed 4 January 2025)

Haraway. D. (2016), *Staying with the trouble: Making kin in the Chthulucene*, Durham: Duke University Press.

McKittrick, K. (2021), *Dear science and other stories*, Durham: Duke University Press.

Plumwood, V. (2003), *Feminism and the mastery of nature*, London: Routledge.

Puig de la Bellacasa, M. (2017), *Matters of care: Speculative ethics in more than human worlds*, Minneapolis: Minnesota University Press.

Singh, N. (2017), 'Becoming a commoner: The commons as sites for affective socio-nature encounters and cobecomings', *Ephemera: Theory & Politics in Organization*, 17 (4): 751–776.

Todd, Z. (2016), 'An indigenous feminist's take on the ontological turn: "Ontology" is just another word for colonialism', *Journal of Historical Sociology*, 29 (1): 4–22.

Tronto, J. (2017), 'There is an alternative: Homines curans and the limits of neoliberalism', *International Journal of Care and Caring*, 1 (1): 27–43.

Tsing, A. (2015), *The mushroom at the end of the world: On the possibility of life in capitalist ruins*, Princeton: Princeton University Press.

Vasudevan, P., M.M. Ramírez, Y. González Mendoza and M. Daigle (2023), 'Storytelling Earth and Body', *Annals of the American Association of Geographers*, 113 (7): 1728–1744, DOI: 10.1080/24694452.2022.2139658.

Wynter, S. (2003), 'Unsettling the coloniality of being/power/truth/freedom: Towards the human, after man, its over-representation – an argument', *CR: The New Centennial Review* 3 (3): 257–337. DOI: 10.1353/ncr.2004.0015

2 Care work: Valuing Social Reproduction

Agarwal, B., R. Venkatachalam and F. Cerniglia (2021), 'Women, pandemics and the Global South: An introductory overview', *Economia Politica* 39: 15–30.

Arora, S., B. Van Dyck, D. Sharma and A. Stirling (2020), 'Control, care, and conviviality in the politics of technology for sustainability', *Sustainability: Science, Practice and Policy* 16 (1): 247–262.

Banfi, L. (2008), 'Lavoro domestico, politiche migratorie e immigrazione filip- pina. Un confronto tra Canada e Italia' (Dometic work and the politics of Filippino migration and immigration: A comparison between Canada and Italy), *Polis* 22: 5–34.

Banks, N. (2020), 'Black women in the United States and unpaid collective work: Theorizing the community as a site of production', *The Review of Black Political Economy* 47 (4): 343–362.

Barca, S. (2024), *Workers of the Earth, labour, ecology and reproduction in the age of climate change*, London: Pluto Press.

Basa, C., V. De Guzman and S. Marchetti (2012), 'International migration and over-indebtedness: The case of Filipino workers in Italy', *IIED – Human Settlements Working Paper*, 36.

Blanco, M. L. and M. G. Cuervo (2021), 'The pandemic as a portal: Policy transformations disputing the new normal'. Development Alternatives with Women for a New Era (DAWN) Discussion Paper No.32. Suva Fiji: DAWN.

Bravo Arias, A. (2022), 'Contested care politics: Perspectives in- against- and-beyond the state in the times of Chilean institutional reconfiguration', *ISS Working Paper*. The Hague: International Institute of Social Studies.

Budlender, D., ed. (2010), *Time use studies and unpaid care work*, London/New York: Routledge.

The Care Collective (2020), *The care manifesto: The politics of interdependence*, London/New York: Verso.

Cirmi Obon, B. (2017), 'Who flies the kite? Argentinean parental leave design: Care penalties for the included and the excluded families', *ISS Working Paper*. The Hague: International Institute of Social Studies.

Collantes, C. (2016), 'Reproductive dilemmas, labour and remittances: Gender and intimacies in Cavite, Philippines', *South East Asia Research* 24 (1): 77–97.

Curty, G. (2020), 'Rethinking capitalism, crisis, and critique: An interview with Nancy Fraser', *Critical Sociology* 46 (7–8): 1327–1337.

DAWN (2022), *DAWN Discussion Papers 2021–2*. Suva, Fiji: DAWN Available online: https://dawnnet.org/discussion-papers/ (Accessed 6 January 2025).

Dengler, C. and M. Lang (2021). 'Commoning care: Feminist degrowth visions for a socio-ecological transformation', *Feminist Economics*, 28 (1): 1–28.

Di Chiro, G. (2019), 'Care not growth: Imagining a subsistence economy for all', *The British Journal of Politics and International Relations*, 21 (20): 303–311.

Ehrenreich, B. and A. Hochschild (2004), *Global woman. Nannies, maids, and sex workers in the new economy*, New York: Holt Paperbacks.

Fine, M. and J. Tronto (2020), 'Care goes viral: Care theory and research confront the global COVID-19 pandemic', 4 (3): 301–309, *International Journal of Care and Caring*, DOI: 10.1332/239788220X15924188322978

Fisher, B. and J. Tronto (1990), 'Toward a feminist theory of care', in E. K. Abel and M. K. Nelson (eds), *Circles of care: Work and identity in women's lives*, 36–54, New York: State University of New York Press.

Folbre, N. (2014), 'Who's cares? A feminist critique of the care economy', Discussions Paper. New York: Rosa Luxemburg Stiftung. Available online: https://www.rosalux.de/fileadmin/rls_uploads/pdfs/sonst_publikationen/folbre_whocares.pdf (Accessed 4 January 2025).

Folbre, N. (2017), *The care penalty and gender inequality*, Amherst: University of Massachusetts.

Fraser, N. (2016), 'Contradictions of capital and care', *New Left Review* 100 (July/August): 99–117.

Harcourt, W., A. Agostino, R. Elmhirst, M. Gomez and P. Kotsila (eds) (2023), *Contours of Feminist Political Ecology*, London: Palgrave.

Hawai'i State Commission on the Status of Women (2020), 'Building bridges, not walking on backs: Hawai'i State Commission on the Status of Women Department of Human Services State of Hawai'i: A feminist economic recovery plan for COVID-19', Available online: https://humanservices.hawaii.gov/wp-content/uploads/2020/04/4.13.20-Final-Cover-D2-Feminist-Economic-Recovery-D1.pdf (Accessed 4 January 2025).

Kabeer, N., S. Razavi and Y. van der Meulen Rodgers (2021). 'Feminist economic perspectives on the COVID-19 pandemic', *Feminist Economics* 27 (1–2): 1–29.

Krasny, E. (2022), *Living with an infected planet: COVID-19, feminism, and the global frontline of care*, Everand E-book.

Lithander, F. E., S. Neumann, E. Tenison, K. Lloyd, T. J. Welsh, J. C. L. Rodrigues, J. P. T. Higgins, L. Scourfield, H. Christensen, V. J. Haunton and E. Henderson (2020), 'COVID-19 in older people: A rapid clinical review', *Age and Ageing*, 49 (4): 501–515. https://doi.org/10.1093/ageing/afaa093

Magat, M. (2004), 'Women breadwinners in the margins: Filipina domestic workers in Rome, Italy', in A. Fauve-Chamoux (ed.), *Domestic service and the formation of European identity. Understanding the globalization of domestic work, 16th–21st centuries*, Bern: Peter Lang.

Marchetti, S. (2016), 'Citizenship and maternalism in migrant domestic labour: Filipina workers and their employers in Amsterdam and Rome', (147–168), in Gullikstad, B. (ed.), *Paid migrant domestic labour in a changing Europe*, DOI: 10.1057/978-1-137-51742-5_7

Mezzadri, A. (2022), 'Social reproduction and pandemic neoliberalism: Planetary crises and the reorganisation of life, work and death', *Organization* 29 (3): 379–400.

Mezzadri, A., S.M. Rai, S. Stevano, D. Alessandrini, H. Bargawi, J. Elias, S. Hassim, S. Kesar, J. Thiyaga Lingham, S. Natile N. Neetha, L. Ossome, P. Raghuram, D. Tsikata and S. Wohl (2025), 'Pluralizing social reproduction approaches', *International Feminist Journal of Politics* (published online 3 February 2025): 1–28. DOI: 10.1080/14616742.2024.2447594

Murphy, M. (2015) 'Unsettling care: Troubling transnational itineraries of care in feminist health practices', *Social Studies of Science* 45 (5): 717–737.

Natile, S. (2022), 'Towards feminist recovery plans policy', *Brief 7*, University of Warwick: Global Centre, Available online: https://warwick.ac.uk/fac/soc/law/research/centres/globe/policybriefs/pb7_towards_feminist_recovery_plans_for_covid19_and_beyond_-_serena_natile_feb22.pdf (Accessed 4 January 2025).

Ojeda, D., N. Padini, D. Rocheleau and J. Emel (2022), 'Feminist ecologies', *Annual Review Enviroment and Resources* 47: 149–171.

Puig de la Bellacasa, M. (2017), *Matters of care. Speculative ethics in more than human worlds*, Minneapolis: Minnesota University Press.

Rai, S. (2024), *Depletion: The human costs of caring*, Oxford: Oxford University Press.

Suchet-Pearson, S., S. Wright, K. Lloyd and L. Burarrwanga with Bawaka Country (2013), 'Caring as country: Towards an ontology of co-becoming in natural resource management', *Asia Pacific Viewpoint* 54 (2): 185–197.

Todaro, R. and I. Arriagada (2020), 'Global care chains', 347–364, in N. Naples (ed.), *Companion to Gender Studies*, Oxford: Wiley-Blackwell.

Tronto, J. (2010), 'Creating caring institutions: Politics, plurality, and purpose', *Ethics and Social Welfare* 4 (2): 158–171.

Tronto, J. (2023) 'Beyond wealth-care: Pandemic dreams for a just and caring future', in M. Duffy, A. Armenia and K. Price-Glynn, *From crisis to catastrophe: Care, COVID, and pathways to change*, New Brunswick: Rutgers University Press.

UN Women (2021), 'Beyond Covid-19: A feminist plan for sustainability and social justice', UN Women Research and Data Section, New York: UN Women. Available online: https://www.unwomen.org/sites/default/files/Headquarters/Attachments/Sections/Library/Publications/2021/Feminist-plan-for-sustainability-and-social-justice-en.pdf (Accessed 4 January 2025).

Vine, M. and J. Tronto (2020), 'Care goes viral: Care theory and research confront the global COVID-19 pandemic', 4 (3): 301–309, *International Journal of Care and Caring*, DOI: 10.1332/239788220X15924188322978

Yeates, N. (2004), 'Global care chains', *International Feminist Journal of Politics* 6 (3): 369–391.

Yeates, N. (2009), *Globalizing care economies and migrant workers: Explorations in global care chains*, New York: Palgrave Macmillan.

Zechner, M. (2015), 'Barcelona en Comú: The city as horizon for radical democracy', *Roar Magazine*. Available online: https://roarmag.org/essays/barcelona-en-comu-guanyem/ (Accessed 4 January 2025).

Zechner, M. (2020), 'Heteropolitics: Refiguring the common and the political', Available online: https://heteropolitics.net/wp-content/uploads/2020/12/Case-Studies-in-Spain.pdf (Accessed 4 January 2025).

Zechner, M. (2021), *Commoning care & collective power: Childcare commons and the micropolitics of municipalism in Barcelona*, Vienna: Transversal Texts.

3 Earthcare: Ecofeminist and Indigenous Approaches to Our Life-worlds

Barca, S., G. Di Chiro, W. Harcourt, I. Iengo, P. Kotsila. S. Kulkarni, I. Leonardelli and C. Sato (2023), 'Caring communities for radical change: What can feminist political ecology bring to degrowth?', 177–206, in W. Harcourt, A. Agostino, R. Elmhirst, M. Gómez and P. Kotsila (eds), *Contours of feminist political ecology*, London: Palgrave Macmillan.

Bawaka Country, S. Wright, S. Suchet-Pearson, K. Lloyd, L. Burarrwanga, R. Ganambarr, M. Ganambarr-Stubbs, B. Ganambarr, D. Maymuru and J. Sweeney. *Co-becoming* (2016), 'Co-becoming Bawaka: Towards a relational understanding of place/space', *Progress in Human Geography* 40(4): 455–475.

Bird Rose, D. (2003), *Report on sharing kinship with nature: How reconciliation is transforming the NSW national parks and wildlife service*, Sydney: National Parks and Wildlife Service, NSW. Available online: https://www.environment.nsw.gov.au/resources/cultureheritage/SharingKinship.pdf (Accessed 6 January 2025).

Bird Rose, D. (2013a), 'Slowly ~ writing into the anthropocene', *TEXT* Special Issue 20: Writing Creates Ecology and Ecology Creates Writing, 6 October: 1–14, https://doi.org/10.52086/001c.28826

Bird Rose, D. (2013b), 'Val Plumwood's philosophical animism: Attentive interactions in the sentient world', *Environmental Humanities* 3: 93–109.

Britten, E. (2023), 'Ocean and Human Health', 297–305, in F. Obaidullah (ed.), *The ocean and us*, Switzerland: Springer Nature.

Chandler, D. and J. Reid (2020), 'Becoming Indigenous: The 'speculative turn' in anthropology and the (re)colonisation of indigeneity', *Postcolonial Studies* 23(4): 1–20.

Cock, J. (1992), 'The World Women's Congress for a Healthy Planet agenda: Empower women for gender equity', *Rural Politics* 12: 63–66, https://doi.org/10.2307/4065479

Dankelman, I. (2010), 'Introduction: Exploring gender, environment and climate change', 1–18, in I. Dankelman (ed.), *Gender, environment and climate change: An introduction*, London: Routledge.

Giakoumi, S., C. Pita, M. Coll, S. Fraschetti, E. Gissi, I. Katara, E. Lloret-Lloret, F. Rossi, M. Portman, V. Stelzenmüller and F. Micheli (2021), 'Persistent gender bias in marine science and conservation calls for action to achieve equity', *Biological Conservation*, 257, 109134, https://doi.org/10.1016/j.biocon.2021.109134

Gibson-Graham, J. K. (2011), 'A feminist project of belonging for the Anthropocene', *Gender, Place and Culture* 18 (1): 1–21.

Hill, R. P. L. Pert, J. Davies, C. J. Robinson, F. Walsh and F. Falco-Mammone (2013), 'Indigenous land management in Australia. Extent, scope, diversity, barriers and success factors', Cairns: CSIRO Ecosystem Sciences.

Kimmerer, R. W. (2013), *Braiding sweetgrass: Indigenous wisdom, scientific knowledge, and the teachings of plants*, Minneapolis: Milkweed Editions.

Kirksey, E. (2021), 'Obituary: Deborah Bird Rose (1946–2018)', *The Asia Pacific Journal of Anthropology* 22 (1): 81–83, DOI: 10.1080/14442213.2020.1867956

Lang, M. (2022), 'Buen vivir as a territorial practice: Building a more just and sustainable life through interculturality', *Sustainability Science* 2022 (4): 1287–1299.

Nakata, S. and S. Maddison (2019), 'New collaborations in old institutional spaces: Setting a new research agenda to transform Indigenous-settler relations', *Australian Journal of Political Science* 54 (3): 407–422, DOI: 10.1080/10361146.2019.1626347

Obaidullah, F. (ed.) (2023), *The ocean and us*, Switzerland: Springer Nature.

Ojeda, D., N. Padini, D. Rocheleau and J. Emel (2022), 'Feminist Ecologies', *Annual Review Enviroment and Resources* 47: 149–171.

Plumwood, V. (2003), *Feminism and the Mastery of Nature*, London: Routledge.

Plumwood, V. (2007), 'A review of Deborah Bird Rose's Reports from a Wild Country: Ethics of Decolonisation', *Australian Humanities Review* 42: 1–4.

Plumwood, V. (2008), *The eye of the crocodile*, Canberra: ANU Press.

Shiva, V. (1988), *Staying alive: Women, ecology and development*, London: Zed Books.

Singh, V. (2021), 'Forward', xviii–xxvii, in D. A. Vakoch (ed.), *Dystopias and utopias on Earth and beyond: Feminist ecocriticism of science fiction*, London: Routledge.

Suchet-Pearson, S., S. Wright, K. Lloyd and L. Burarrwanga with Bawaka Country (2013), 'Caring as Country: Towards an ontology of co-becoming in natural resource management', *Asia Pacific Viewpoint* 54 (2): 185–197.

Turhan, E. (2022), 'Keeping the world alive and healthy: The radical realism of the forces of reproduction – An interview with Stefania Barca', *Undisciplined Environments*, 25 January 2022. Available online: https://undisciplinedenvironments.org/author/undisciplined-environments/ (Accessed 4 January 2025)

Watson, I. (2018), 'Aboriginal relationships to the natural world: Colonial "protection" of human rights and the environment', *Journal of Human Rights and the Environment* 9 (2): 119–140.

Whyte, K. (2018), 'Settler colonialism, ecology, and environmental injustice', *Environment and Society* 9 (1): 125–144.

Yumie Aoki Inoue, C. (2018), 'Worlding the study of global environmental politics in the anthropocene: Indigenous voices from the Amazon', *Global Environmental Politics* 18 (4): 25–42.

4 Caring about Having Babies: Reproductive Rights and Population Ethics

Bhatia, R., J. Sasser, D. Ojeda, A. Hendrixson, S. Nadimpally and E. E. Foley (2020), 'A feminist exploration of "populationism": Engaging contemporary forms of population control', *Gender, Place & Culture* 27 (3): 333–350, https://doi.org/10.1080/0966369X.2018.1553859

Carrington, D. (10 May 2024), '"I am starting to panic about my child's future": climate scientists wary of starting families climate crisis', *The Guardian*. Available online: https://www.theguardian.com/environment/article/2024/may/10/climate-scientists-starting-families-children?CMP=Share (Accessed 4 January 2025).

Coole, D. (2013), 'Too many bodies? The return and disavowal of the population question', *Environmental Politics* 22 (2): 195–215, https://doi.org/10.1080/09644016.2012.730268

Clarke, A. E. and D. Haraway (2018), *Making kin not population: Reconceiving generations*, Chicago: Prickly Paradigm Press.

Di Chiro, G. (2008), 'Living environmentalisms: Coalition politics, social reproduction, and environmental justice', *Environmental Politics* 17 (2): 276–298.

Fenner, M. and W. Harcourt (2023), 'Debating population in and beyond feminist political ecology', 231–257, in W. Harcourt, A. Agostino, R. Elmhirst, M. Gómez and P. Kotsila (eds), *Contours of Feminist Political Ecology*, London: Palgrave Macmillan.

Haraway, D. (2015), 'Anthropocene, capitalocene, plantationocene, Chthulucene: Making kin', *Environmental Humanities* 6 (1): 159–165, https://doi.org/10.1215/22011919-3615934

Haraway, D. (2016), *Staying with the trouble: Making kin in the Chthulucene*, Durham: Duke University Press.

Haraway, D. (2017), 'Response to life with Ms Cayenne Pepper', *London Review of Books* 39 (13). Available online: https://www.lrb.co.uk/the-paper/v39/n13/letters (Accessed 28 July 2022).

Haraway, D. (2018), 'Making kin in the Chthulucene: Reproducing multispecies justice', 67–100, in D. Haraway and A. Clarke (eds), *Making kin not population: Reconceiving generations*, Chicago: Prickly Paradigm Press.

Harcourt, W. (2009), *Body politics in development: Critical debates in gender and development*, London: Zed Books.

Harcourt, W. (2020), 'Unravelling the 'P' word in environment and development', *Development and Change* 51 (6): 1628–1639, https://doi.org/10.1111/dech.12619

Hartmann, B. (1995), *Reproductive rights and wrongs: The global politics of population control*, Boston: South End Press.

Hartmann, B. (1998), 'Population, environment and security: A new trinity', *Environment and Urbanization* 10 (2): 113–128.

Howard, L. (2022), 'When global problems come home: Engagement with climate change within the intersecting affective spaces of parenting and activism', *Emotion, Space and Society* 44 (August): 1–8, https://doi.org/10.1016/j.emospa.2022.100894xy2

Jolly, J. (2016), 'Forbidden wombs and transnational reproductive justice', *Meridians: Feminism, Race, Transnationalism* 15 (1): 166–188.

Lewis, S. (2017), 'Less "population" talk, more kin-making: On Manchester's B!RTH festival', *Feminist Review* 117: 193–199.

Mehta, L. (ed.) (2019), *The limits to scarcity: Contesting the politics of allocation*, London: Earthscan.

Ojala, M., A. Cunsolo, C. Ogunbode and J. Middleton (2021), 'Anxiety, worry, and grief in a time of environmental and climate crisis: A narrative review', *Annual Review of Environment and Resources* 46: 35–58.

Ojeda, D., J. Sasser and E. Lunstrum (2019), 'Malthus's specter and the anthropocene', *Gender, Place and Culture* 27 (3): 316–332, https://doi.org/10.1080/0966369X.2018.1553858

Ray, S. J. (March 2021), 'Climate anxiety is an overwhelmingly white phenomenon', *Scientific American*. Available online: https://www.scientificamerican.com/article/the-unbearable-whiteness-of-climate-anxiety/ (Accesed 5 January 2025).

Sasser, J. S. (2014), 'From darkness into light: Race, population, and environmental advocacy', *Antipode* 46 (5): 1240–1257, https://doi.org/10.1111/anti.12029.

Sasser, J. S. (2018), *On infertile ground: Population control and women's rights in the era of climate change*, New York: New York University Press.

Sasser, J. S. (2024), 'At the intersection of climate justice and reproductive justice', *WIREs Climate Change* 15 (1): 1–13, https://doi.org/10.1002/wcc.860.

Schneider-Mayerson, M. and K. L. Leong (2020), 'Eco-reproductive concerns in the age of climate change', *Climatic Change* 163: 1007–1023, https://doi.org/10.1007/s10584-020-02923-y

Schultz, S. (2021), 'The neo-Malthusian reflex in climate politics: Technocratic, right wing and feminist references', *Australian*

Feminist Studies 36 (110): 485–502, https://doi.org/10.1080/08164649.20 21.1995847

Silliman, J. and Y. King (1999), *Dangerous intersections: Feminist perspectives on population, environment, and development*, Boston: South End Press.

Subramaniam, B. (2018), '"Overpopulation" is not the problem', in Feminism section of the website Public Books. Available online: https://www.publicbooks.org/overpopulation-is-not-the-problem/ (Accessed 4 January 2025).

Wilson, K. (2017), 'Re-centring "race" in development: Population policies and global capital accumulation in the era of the SDGs', *Globalizations* 14 (3): 432–449.

5 Interspecies Care: Learning with the More-than-Human

Adams, C. J. (1990), *The sexual politics of meat: A feminist-vegan critical theory*, NY: Continuum.

Adams, C. J. (1991), 'Ecofeminism and the eating of animals', *Hypatia* 6: 125–145, https://doi.org/10.1111/j.1527-2001.1991.tb00213.x

Bear, C. (2021), 'Making insects tick: Responsibility, attentiveness and care in edible insect farming', *Environment and Planning E: Nature and Space* 4 (3): 1010–1030, https://doi.org/10.1177/ 2514848620945321

Berne, P. and V. Raditz (31 July 2019), 'To survive climate catastrophe, look to queer and disabled folks', *Yes! Magazine*. Available online: https://www.yesmagazine.org/opinion/2019/07/31/climate-change-queer-disabled-organizers (Accessed 5 January 2025).

Chao, S. (2022), *In the shadow of the palms: More-than-human becomings in West Papua*, Durham: Duke University Press.

Chao, S., K. Bolender and E. Kirksey (eds) (2022), *The promise of multispecies justice*, Durham: Duke University Press.

Chen, M. Y. (2012), *Animacies: Biopolitics, racial mattering, and queer affect*, Durham: Duke University Press.

Chen, M. Y. (2023), *Intoxicated: Race, disability, and chemical intimacy across empire*, Durham: Duke University Press.

Cielemęcka, O. and C. Åsberg (2019), 'Toxic embodiment and feminist environmental humanities', *Environmental Humanities* 11 (1): 101–107, DOI:10.1215/22011919-7349433

Desai, S. and H. Smith (2018), 'Kinship across species: Learning to care for nonhuman others', *Feminist Review* 118: 41–60.

Di Chiro, G. (2010), 'Polluted politics? Confronting toxic discourse, sex panic, and eco normativity', 199–230, in C. Mortimer-Sandilands and B. Erickson (eds), *Queer ecologies: Sex, nature, politics, desire*, Bloomington: Indiana University Press.

van Dooren, T. (2014), 'Care', Living Lexicon for the Environmental Humanities, *Environmental Humanities* 5: 291–294. Available online: https://www.environmentandsociety.org/sites/default/files/key_docs/environmental_humanities-2014-van_dooren-291-4.pdf (Accessed 5 January 2025).

Fernando, J. L. (2020), 'From the Virocene to the Lovecene epoch: multispecies justice as critical praxis for Virocene disruptions and vulnerabilities', *Journal of Political Ecology* 27 (1): 685–731, https://doi.org/10.2458/v27i1.23816

Gaard, G. (1993), *Ecofeminism: Women, animals, nature*, Philadelphia, PA: Temple University Press.

Gaard, G. (2011), 'Ecofeminism revisited: Rejecting essentialism and re-placing species in a material feminist environmentalism', *Feminist Formations* 23 (2): 26–53.

Gordon-Nembhard, J. (2023). 'Black political economy, solidarity economics, and liberation: Towards an economy of caring and abundance', *Review of Radical Political Economics* 55 (4): 525–538.

Gumbs, A. P. (2020), *Undrowned: Black feminist lessons from marine mammals*, Chico, CA: AK Press.

Hamilton, J. M. and A. Neimanis (2018), 'Composting feminisms and environmental humanities', *Environmental Humanities* 10 (2): 501–527, https://doi.org/10.1215/22011919-7156859

Haraway, D. (2011), 'Speculative fabulations for technoculture's generations: Taking care of unexpected country', *Australian Humanities*, Issue 50. Available online: https://australianhumanitiesreview.org/2011/05/01/speculative-fabulations-for-technocultures-generations-taking-care-of-unexpected-country/ (Accessed 5 January 2025).

Harcourt, W. and X. Argüello Calle (2022), 'Embodying cyberspace: Making the personal political in digital places', 83–112, in W. Harcourt, K. van den Berg, C. Dupuis and J. Gaybor (eds), *Feminist methodologies*, London: Palgrave Macmillan.

Ives, S. (2019), '"More-than-human" and "less-than-human": Race, botany, and the challenge of multispecies ethnography', *Catalyst: Feminism, Theory, Technoscience* 5 (2): 1–5.

Krzywoszynska, A. (2019), 'Caring for soil life in the Anthropocene: The role of attentiveness in more-than-human ethics', *Transactions of the Institute of British Geographers* 44: 661–675.

Krzywoszynska, A. and G. Marchesi (2020), 'Toward a relational materiality of soils: Introduction', *Environmental Humanities* 12 (1): 190–204, https://doi.org/10.1215/22011919-8142297

Liljeström, M. (2015), 'Affect', in L. Disch and M. Hawkesworth (eds), *The Oxford handbook of feminist theory*, Oxford Handbooks' 16–38, https://doi.org/10.1093/oxfordhb/9780199328581.013.3

McRuer, R. (2006), *Crip theory: Cultural signs of queerness and disability*, New York: New York University Press.

Mol, A., I. Mosser and J. Pols (2010), 'Care: Putting practice into theory', 7–25, in A. Mol, I. Mosser and J. Pols (eds), *Care in practice: On tinkering in clinics, homes and farms*. New Brunswick, NJ: Verlag.

Neimanis, A. and L. McLauchlan (2022), 'Composting (in) the Gender Studies classroom: Growing feminisms for climate changing pedagogies', *Curriculum Inquiry* 52 (2): 218–234.

Oliver, C. (2024), *What is veganism for?*, Bristol: Bristol University Press.

Piepzna-Samarasinha, L. L. (2020), 'Still dreaming wild disability justice dreams at the end of the world', 250–261, in A. Wong (ed.), *Disability visibility: First-person stories from the twenty-first century*, New York: Vintage Books.

Pitt, H. (2018), 'Questioning care cultivated through connecting with more-than-human communities', *Social & Cultural Geography* 19 (2): 253–274. https://doi.org/10.1080/14649365.2016.1275753.

Pratt, S. (2019) 'Care, toxics and being prey: I want to be good food for others', *Australian Feminist Studies* 34 (102): 437–453, DOI: 10.1080/08164649.2019.1702873

Puig de la Bellacasa, M. (2010), *Matters of care: Speculative ethics in more than human worlds*, Minneapolis: Minnesota University Press.

Sandilands, C. (2021), 'Plant/s matter', *Women's Studies* 50 (8): 776–783, DOI: 10.1080/00497878.2021.1983433

Tsing, A. (2010), 'Arts of inclusion, or, how to love a mushroom,' *Manoa* 22 (2): 191–203.

Tsing, A. (2015), *The mushroom at the end of the world: On the possibility of life in capitalist ruins*, Princeton: Princeton University Press.

Turner, B., A. Hill and J. Abramovic (2024), 'Learning with compost: Digging down into food waste, urban soils and community', *Local Environment* (Online version July 2024): 1–15, https://doi.org/10.1080/1 3549839.2024.2380853

Twine, R. (2024), *The climate crisis and other animals*, Sydney: Sydney University Press.

Ureta, S., M. Llona, D. Rodríguez-Oroz, D. Valenzuela, C. Trujillo-Espinoza, C. Guiñez, A. Rebolledo, M. J. Maiza and C. Rodríguez Beltrán (2022), 'Nuestros Suelos: Exploring new forms of public engagement with polluted soils', *Journal of Science Communication* 21 (01): 1–13, https://doi.org/10.22323/2.21010801

Wandersee, J. H. and E. E. Schussler (1999), 'Preventing plant blindness', *The American Biology Teacher* 61: 82–86, DOI: 10.2307/4450624

Yee, K. and E. L. Sharp (2023), 'Complexities of care in insect-human relations', *New Zealand Geographer* 79 (2): 86–96, https://doi.org/10.1111/nzg.12369

6 Caring Communities: Building Reciprocity through Degrowth, Community Economies and Radical Care

Bauwens, M., V. Kostakis and A. Pazaitis (2019), *Peer to peer: The commons manifesto*, London: University of Westminster Press. Available online: library.oapen.org/bitstream/id/2e3f561d-b1f5-4e7c-8da3-ccab0f00501d/ UWP-033-REVISED.pdf (Accessed 5 January 2025).

Akbulut, B. (2021), 'Degrowth', *Rethinking Marxism* 33 (1): 98–110, DOI: 10.1080/08935696.2020.1847014

Burke, B. J. and B. W. Shear (2014), 'Introduction: Engaged scholarship for non-capitalist political ecologies', in special section 'Non-capitalist political ecologies', *Journal of Political Ecology* 21: 127–221.

Clement, F., W. Harcourt, D. Joshi and C. Sato (2019), 'Feminist political ecologies of the commons and commoning', *International Journal of the Commons* 13 (1): 1–15.

De Angelis, M. (2017), 'Grounding social revolution: Elements for a systems theory of commoning', 213–256, in G. Ruivenkamp and A. Hilton (eds), *Perspectives on commoning: Autonomist principles and practices*, London: Zed Books.

Day, E. (2021), 'Working in the Trouble and Jane Bennett's middle ground: Animating creative projects in the Australian Anthropocene', 185–195, in J. Millner and G. Coombs (eds), *Care ethics and art*, London: Routledge. DOI: 10.4324/9781003167556-18

Di Chiro, G. (2019), 'Care not growth: Imagining a subsistence economy for all', *The British Journal of Politics and International Relations* 21 (2): 303–311.

Dombroski, K. (2024a), *Caring for life: A postdevelopment politics of infant hygiene*, Minneapolis: University of Minnesota Press.

Dombroksi, K. (2024b), 'The nappy revolution', *Revaluing Care Blog*, 18 November 2024. Available online: https://www.revaluingcare.org/the-nappy-revolution/ (Accessed 5 January 2025).

Dombroski, K., S. Healy and K. McKinnon (2019), 'Care-full community economies', 99–115, in C. Bauhardt and W. Harcourt (eds), *Feminist Political Ecology and the Economics of Care*, London: Routledge.

Edelman, E. A. (2020), 'Beyond resilience: Trans coalitional activism as radical self-care', *Social Text* 38 (1 (142)): 109–130.

Federici, S. and G. Caffentzis (2014), 'Commons against and beyond capitalism', *Community Development Journal* 49 (1): 92–105.

Feola, G., A. AlSalem, O. Alakavuklar and Y. Rahmouni Elidrissi (2025), 'Prospects for coalition building across difference: Discourse similarity, complementarity, or equivalence?', *International Journal of Politics, Culture, and Society*, Published online 27 March 2025, https://doi.org/10.1007/s10767-025-09512-w

Fitz, A. and E. Krasny (eds) (2019), *Critical care: Architecture and urbanism for a broken planet*. Architekturzentrum Wien: MIT Press Direct. https://doi.org/10.7551/mitpress/12273.001.0001

Gibson-Graham, J. K. (2006), *A postcapitalist politics*, Minneapolis and London: University of Minnesota Press.

Gibson-Graham, J. K., J. Cameron and S. Healy (2013), *Take back the economy: An ethical guide for transforming our communities*, Minneapolis: University of Minnesota Press.

Gibson-Graham, J. K. and K. Dombroski (eds) (2020), *The handbook of diverse economies*, Cheltenham UK: Edward Elgar.

Haynes, R. (2021), 'Threads of resistance feminist activism, collaborative making and care ethics', 119–130, in J. Millner and G. Coombs (eds), *Care ethics and art*, London: Routledge.

Hecker, S. and M. Taddicken (2022). 'Deconstructing citizen science: A framework on communication and interaction using the concept of roles', *JCOM* 21 (01), A07, https://doi.org/10.22323/2.21010207

Hine, D. (2023), *At work in the ruins: Finding our place in the time of science, climate change, pandemics and all the other emergencies*, London: Chelsea Green Publishing.

Hobart, K. H. J. and T. Kneese (2020), 'Radical care: Survival strategies for uncertain times', *Social Text* 142, 38 (1): 1–16.

Iengo, I. (2025). 'Naples, 2032. Visionary fragments of the eco-transfeminist city', *Antipode: A radical journal of geography* 57(3): 996–1016. https://doi.org/10.1111/anti.70000

Just Transitions Coordinating Team (2022), *Policy brief on care work in the Just Transitions*, Geneva: UNRISD. Available online: https://cdn.unrisd.org/assets/library/briefs/pdf-files/2024/pb-2024-jtc-care-work-just-transitions.pdf (Accessed 5 January 2025).

Kaul, S., B. Akbulut, F. Demaria, and J-F. Gerber (2022), 'Alternatives to sustainable development: What can we learn from the pluriverse in practice?', *Sustainability Science* 17: 1149–1158.

Klein, E., J. Hunt, Z. Staines, Y. Dinku, C. Brown, K. Glynn-Braun and M. Yap, advised by M. Murray and B. Williamson (2023), *Caring about Care Wiyi Yani U Thangani*, Canberra: The Australian National University. Available online: https://wiyiyaniuthangani.humanrights.gov.

au/sites/default/files/2024-03/Caring%20about%20Care%20Report%20 2024.pdf (Accessed 5 January 2025).
La Via Campesina (2021), 'The path of peasant and popular feminism in La Via Campesina'. Available online: https://viacampesina.org/en/publication-the-path-of-peasant-and-popular-feminism-in-la-via-campesina/ (Accessed 5 January 2025).
Murphy, M. (2015), 'Unsettling care: Troubling transnational itineraries of care in feminist health practices', *Social Studies of Science* 45 (5): 717–737.
Nakamura, N. and C. Sato (2023), 'More-than-human commoning through women's Kokorozashi business for collective well-being: A Case from aging and depopulating rural Japan', *International Journal of the Commons* 17 (1): 125–140.
Nieto-Romero, M., G. García-López, P. Swagemakers and B. Bock (2023), 'Becoming a care-tizen: Contributing to democracy through forest commoning', *International Journal of the Commons* 17 (1): 271–287.
Non Una di Meno (2020), 'Life beyond the pandemic', trans. E. Gainsforth and M. Tola, *Interface, a Journal for and about Social Movements, Sharing Stories of Struggles* (May): 1–6. Available online: https://www.interfacejournal.net/wp-content/uploads/2020/05/Non-Una-Di-Meno-Roma.pdf (Accessed 5 January 2025).
Phillips, C. (2021), 'Stand your ground: Global solidarity through creative care', 268–278, in J. Millner and G. Coombs (eds), *Care ethics and art*, London: Routledge. DOI:10.4324/9781003167556-26
Piepzna-Samarasinha, L. L. (2018), *Care work: Dreaming disability justice*, Vancouver: Arsenal Pulp Press.
Portocarrero Lacayo, A. V. (2024), 'Care is the new radical: Food and climate approaches from a peasant feminist perspective', *The Journal of Peasant Studies*, published online February 2024, DOI: 10.1080/03066150.2024.2306987
Puig de la Bellacasa, M. (2011), 'Matters of care in technoscience: Assembling neglected things', *Social Studies of Science* 41 (1): 85–106.
Reese, A. M. and S. A. Johnson (2022), 'We all we got: Urban black ecologies of care and mutual aid', *Environment and Society* 13 (1): 27–42. http://dx.doi.org/10.3167/ares.2022.130103

Rübner Hansen, B. and M. Zechner (2020), 'Careless networks? Social media, care and reproduction in the web of life', *Spheres: Journal for Digital Cultures* 6, Summer: 1–12, DOI: 10.25969/mediarep/13851

Sató, C. and J. M. Soto Alarcón (2019), 'Toward a postcapitalist feminist political ecology's approach to the commons and commoning', *International Journal of the Commons* 13 (1): 36–61.

Schwenke, C. (2018), *Self-ish: A transgender awakening*, Pasadena, CA: Red Hen Press.

Singh, N. M. (2022), 'The nonhuman turn or a re-turn to animism? Valuing life along and beyond capital', *Dialogues in Human Geography* 12 (1): 84–89.

Solnit, R. (2024), 'Difficult is not the same as impossible', *The Beautiful Truth*, Available online: https://thebeautifultruth.org/world/difficult-is-not-the-same-as-impossible/ (Accessed 21 May 2025).

Tola, M. (2017), 'Species, nature, and the politics of the common: From Virno to Simondon', *The South Atlantic Quarterly* 116 (2): 237–255.

Tronto, J. (2019) 'Caring architecture', 26–32 in A. Fitz and E. Krasny (eds), *Critical care: Architecture and urbanism for a broken planet*. Architekturzentrum Wien: MIT Press Direct. https://doi.org/10.7551/mitpress/12273.003.0004

Zechner, M. (2022), 'Commoning vulnerability? Towards a radical politics of Earthcare', 'After extractivism', *Berliner Gazette*. Available online: https://berlinergazette.de/commoning-vulnerability-towards-a-radical-politics-of-earthcare/ (Accessed 5 January 2025).

Zwarteveen, M., C. Domínguez-Guzmán, M. Kuper, A. Saidani, J. Kemerink-Seyoum, F. Cleaver, H. Kulkarni, L. Bossenbroek, H. Ftouhi, A. Verzijl, U. Aslekar, Z. Kadiri, T. Chitata, I. Leonardelli, S. Kulkarni and S. Bhat (2024), 'Caring for groundwater: How care can expand and transform groundwater governance', *International Journal of the Commons* 18 (1): 384–396, DOI: https://doi.org/10.5334/ijc.1350

7 Connecting with Care: Pedagogies for Transformation

Aguam, J. (2022), *No country for eight-spot butterflies*, Westminster, Maryland: Astra Publishing House.

Arora, S., B. Van Dyck, D. Sharma and A. Stirling (2020), 'Control, care, and conviviality in the politics of technology for sustainability', *Sustainability: Science, Practice and Policy* 16 (1): 247–262, DOI: 10.1080/15487733.2020.1816687

Barca, S., G. Di Chiro, W. Harcourt, I. Iengo, P. Kotsila, S. Kulkarni, I. Leonardelli and C. Sato (2023), 'Caring communities for radical change: What can feminist political ecology bring to degrowth?', 177–206, in W. Harcourt, A. Agostino, R. Elmhirst, M. Gómez and P. Kotsila (eds), *Contours of feminist political ecology*, Palgrave Macmillan, https://doi.org/10.1007/978-3-031-20928-4_8

Carillo Rowe, A. (2005), 'Be longing: Toward a feminist politics of relation', *National Women's Studies Association Journal* 17 (2) (Summer): 15–46, https://www.jstor.org/stable/431712

Carillo Rowe, A. (2008), *Power lines: On the subject of feminist alliances*, Durham: Duke University Press.

Cancar, A. (2023), 'On creating spaces of unlearning in convivial thinking', 7 November. Available online: https://convivialthinking.org/index.php/2023/11/07/on-creating-spaces-of-unlearning/ (Accessed 5 January 2025)

Cavé, D. (2024), 'Learning to "sit in the fire": Staying with the discomfort of transformative learning', *Studies in the Education of Adults*, published online November 2024: 1–18, https://doi.org/10.1080/02660830.2024.2427435

Di Chiro, G. (2006), 'Teaching urban ecology: Environmental studies and the pedagogy of intersectionality', *Feminist Teacher* 16 (2): 98–109, http://www.jstor.org/stable/40545983

Elmhirst, R. and B. Resurrección (2021), *Negotiating gender expertise in environment and development: Voices from feminist political ecology*, London: Routledge.

Escobar, A. (2024) 'Planetary universalisms / Planetary terricide: A pluriversal perspective'. Talk given at the Berggruen Institute Conference 'What is new philosophy for a multipolar world', 21–22 June 2024, held at Palazzo Diedo, Venice. Citations taken from a 16-page copy of the talk shared in word format by the author. For information on the Conference see: https://berggruen.org/projects/universalism (Accessed 5 January 2025).

Goodman, A. (2021), 'Carefull reading: Towards a speculative practice of study in the university', 158–172, in J. Miller and G. Coombes (eds), *Care ethics and art*, London: Routledge.

Gibson-Graham, J. K. and G. Roelvink (2009), 'An economic ethics for the Anthropocene', *Antipode* 41 (1): 320–346, DOI: 10.1111/j.1467-8330.2009.00728.x

Harcourt, W. (2017), 'The making and unmaking of development: Using Post-Development as a tool in teaching development studies', *Third World Quarterly* 38 (12): 2703–2718, https://doi.org/10.1080/01436597.2017.1315300

Harcourt, W. (2018), 'People and personal projects: A rejoinder on the challenge of teaching development studies', *Third World Quarterly* 39 (11): 2203–2205.

Harcourt, W. (2019), 'Feminist political ecology practices of worlding: Art, commoning and the politics of hope in the classroom', *International Journal of the Commons* 13 (1): 153–174, https://doi.org/10.18352/ijc.929/

Hernández, K., J. M. Rubis, N. Theriault, Z. Todd, A. Mitchell, B. Country, L. Burarrwanga, R. Ganambarr, M. Ganambarr-Stubbs, B. Ganambarr, D. Maymuru, S. Suchet-Pearson, K. Lloyd and S. Wright (2021), 'The Creatures Collective: Manifestings', *Environment and Planning E: Nature and Space* 4 (3): 838–863, https://doi.org/10.1177/2514848620938316

hooks, b. (1994), *Teaching to Transgress*, New York: Routledge.

Icaza, R. and Z. Sheik (2023), 'When we couldn't breathe: (Our) stories from the margins', *Globalizations* 20 (2): 201–207, DOI: 10.1080/14747731.2023.2184169.

Kapoor, I. (2023), 'Decolonising development studies', *Review of International Studies* 49 (3): 346–355, DOI: 10.1017/S026021052300013X

Kimmerer, R. W. (2013), 'The rights of the land', *Orion Magazine*. Available online: https://orionmagazine.org/article/the-rights-of-the-land/ (Accessed 5 January 2025).

Kothari, A. (2024), 'VIKALP SANGAM – A decade of exploration on alternatives in India', *Kafila*. Available online: https://kafila.online/2024/09/04/vikalp-sangam-a-decade-of-exploration-on-alternatives-in-india-ashish-kothari/ (Accessed 21 May 2025).

Lang, M. (2022), 'Buen vivir as a territorial practice: Building a more just and sustainable life through interculturality', *Sustainability Science* 17: 1287–1299, https://doi.org/10.1007/s11625-022-01130-1

Lewartowska, E. and L. Riisgaard (2024), 'Scaling out a pluriversality of alternative futures: The case of Vikalp Sangam', *Radical Ecological Democracy*, 17 November. Available online: https://radicalecologicaldemocracy.org/scaling-out-a-pluriversality-of-alternative-futures-the-case-of-vikalp-sangam/ (Accessed 5 January 2025).

Mukhopadhyay, R. (2023), 'Relational care and ordinary repair in diverse craft economies', *Asia Pacific Viewpoint*: 1–7. Available online: https://onlinelibrary.wiley.com/doi/epdf/10.1111/apv.12390 (Accessed 5 January 2025).

Nagar, R., I. Meier and A. Spathopoulou (2023), 'Refusals, radical vulnerability, and hungry translations – a conversation with Richa Nagar', *Fennia* 201 (2): 266–272.

Ojeda, D., P. Nirmal, D. Rocheleau and J. Emel (2022), 'Feminist ecologies', *Annual Review of Environment and Reseources* 47: 149–171, https://doi.org/10.1146/annurev-environ-112320-092246

Pereira, L., G. Di Chiro and I. L. Rigell (2018), 'Situating sustainability against displacement: Building campus-community collaboratives for environmental justice from the ground up', 76–101, in J. Sze (ed.), *Sustainability: Approaches to environmental justice and social power*, New York: NYU Press.

Smith, M. (2011), 'Dis(appearance): Earth, ethics and apparently (in)significant others', *Australian Humanities Review*, Special Issue 'Unloved Others: Death of the Disregarded in the Time of Extinctions', edited by Deborah Bird Rose and Thom van Dooren, 50: 23–44.

Solnit, R. (9 November 2024), 'Authoritarians like Trump love fear, defeatism, surrender. Do not give them what they want', *The Guardian*. Available online: https://www.theguardian.com/world/2024/nov/09/authoritarians-like-trump-love-fear-defeatism-surrender-do-not-give-them-what-they-want (Accessed 5 January 2025).

Suchet-Pearson, S., S. Wright, K. Lloyd and L. Burarrwanga including Bawaka Country (2013), 'Caring as country: Towards an ontology of co-becoming in natural resource management', *Asia Pacific Viewpoint* 54 (2): 185–197.

Sultana, F. (2022), 'Commentary: "Resplendent care-full climate revolutions"', *Political Geography* 99, Article: 102785, https://doi.org/10.1016/j.polgeo.2022.102785

Sundberg, J. (2014), 'Decolonizing posthumanist geographies', *Cultural Geographies* 21 (1): 33–47.

Tall Bear, K. (2019) 'Caretaking relations, not American dreaming', *Kalfou: A Journal of Comparative and Relational Ethnic Studies* 6 (1): 24–41.

Terry, N., A. Castro, B. Chibwe, G. Karuri-Sebina, C. Savu and L. Pereira (2023), 'Inviting a decolonial praxis for future imaginaries of nature: Introducing the Entangled Time Tree', *Environmental Science and Policy* 151, published online January 2024, 103615, https://doi.org/10.1016/j.envsci.2023.103615

Tronto, J. (2013), 'Democratic caring and global responsibilities for care', A Paper prepared for Presentation at the Annual Meeting of the Western Political Science Association, Hollywood, CA, 28–30 March 2013. Available online: https://www.wpsanet.org/papers/docs/Tronto%20WPSA%20paper%202013.pdf (Accessed 5 January 2025).

Tronto, J. (2017), 'There is an alternative: Homines curans and the limits of Neoliberalism', *International Journal of Care and Caring* 1 (1): 27–43.

Truscott, R. and S. M. Khoo (2024), 'On the menu: Academic managerialism and critical theory', *Irish Journal of Sociology* 32 (3): 285–303, https://doi.org/10.1177/07916035241295893

Turner, B., A. Hill and J. Abramovic (2024), 'Learning with compost: Digging down into food waste, urban soils and community', *Local Environment: The International Journal of Justice and Sustainability*, published online July 2024, DOI: 10.1080/13549839.2024.2380853

Walsh, C. (2022), *On decoloniality: Rising up, living on*, Durham: Duke University Press.

Yazzie, M. K. (2023), 'We must make kin to get free: Reflections on #nobanonstolenland in Turtle Island', *Gender, Place and Culture* 30 (4): 596–604.

8 Epilogue

Gregoratti, C., M. Linnell and M. A. Caretta (2024) 'Resilience: Why should we think with care?', *Global Social Challenges Journal* (early view), 1–9, DOI: 10.1332/27523349Y2024D000000033

Harcourt, W. (2023) 'The ethics and politics of care: Reshaping economic thinking and practice', *Review of Political Economy* (1–17), https://doi.org/10.1080/09538259.2023.2241395

Harvey, S. (2024) *Orbital*, London, Grove Press.

Index

Alternative economics 129
Anthropocentricism 62

Barca, Stefania 49, 59, 60, 61, 156, 181
Bawaka Country 70, 71, 72, 180
Bird Rose, Deborah 55, 64–69, 163, 176

Capitalism 13, 28, 50, 70, 88, 108, 114, 124, 133, 134, 147, 163, 175, 181
Care crises 38, 50–51, 84, 134–135, 142–143, 178
Care labour 4, 7–8, 24, 32, 35, 37–39, 43, 45, 47, 53, 61, 87, 132, 135, 138, 140–141
Chao, Sophie 18, 107–108
Chen, Mel 109–110
Childcare 9–10, 36, 46–48, 124, 131, 141
Class 4, 9, 15, 18, 21–22, 36–38, 41–42, 59, 83–84, 87, 90, 91, 95–96, 109–110, 140, 149–154, 159, 162, 165
Climate change 2, 16, 27, 49–52, 59–60, 75, 79–80, 84–95, 102–103, 120, 129, 136–140, 149–150, 175
Colonialism 13–14, 38, 59, 66, 72, 85, 90, 107, 112, 134, 152, 162, 165, 183
Commoning 21, 28, 47, 119, 124, 129–135, 143, 159
Communities 8–9, 13, 15, 18–23, 36, 38, 45, 48, 50–53, 59–60, 65, 70, 72–73, 87–91, 94–96, 102, 105, 106, 112–114, 118–145, 159, 161–168, 177
Community economies 21, 25, 28, 118, 124–129, 135, 145, 178, 182
Conviviality 133, 135, 159
Cosmologies 133, 136, 162
Country (indigenous Australian meaning) 66, 70–72, 75, 138–139, 163, 180

Covid-19 pandemic 2, 11, 26, 31, 33–38, 40, 45, 49, 50–54, 120–124, 141, 155, 178
Crip Theory 110–114, 142, 156, 175, 176

Death 33, 34, 62–63, 66–67, 107–110, 113, 116–118, 142
Decolonial 13, 25, 111, 120, 162, 171
Degrowth 21, 25, 28, 118–124, 135, 140, 145, 178, 181–182.
Development 3, 10, 19, 21–26, 44–45, 56–57, 90, 102, 118, 127–128, 136, 144, 146, 148–158, 161–171, 182
Di Chiro, Giovanna 14, 18, 90, 109, 114, 120, 135, 156–157, 180
Digital technologies 164, 173, 177
Disability 109–114, 117–119, 135, 140–141, 176
Dombroski, Kelly 21, 126–131, 145, 148, 178, 179
Domestic labour 35, 37, 43, 45, 140
van Dooren, Thomas 106–107

Earthcare 14, 27, 54–56, 66–68, 72, 75–77, 159
Earth labour 24, 135, 140, 141
Earthothers 11, 12, 14, 16, 23–24, 27, 55, 62–76, 180
Ecofeminist 12, 14, 27, 57, 61, 64, 109, 114, 117, 156, 159, 181
Ecology 13, 14, 25, 27, 28, 60, 62, 65, 67, 73, 80, 97, 101, 104, 136, 149, 163, 169, 171, 175, 180, 181
Education 10, 18, 22, 76, 111, 136, 146, 148–152, 158–159
Emotions 26, 62, 70–72, 94–96, 122, 149, 156, 164, 167

Environmental justice 18, 25, 27, 55, 57, 61, 65, 73, 88, 90–92, 95, 109, 111, 114, 122, 129, 135, 140, 155–156, 168, 174, 176
Escobar, Arturo 161, 163, 182
Ethics of care 11, 62, 70–72, 79, 93, 100, 104–107, 110, 113, 118, 120, 131, 137, 142, 161, 171, 174

Federici, Silvia 130, 178
Feminism 6, 13, 14, 20, 26–27, 46–49, 76, 80, 91, 97, 112–113, 120, 136, 144, 151, 160, 173, 175, 178
Feminist methodology 1, 25, 105, 156
Feminist movements 19, 27–28, 47, 58, 75, 95, 119, 135, 161, 165, 173
Feminist political ecology 13–14, 25, 27, 101, 136, 169
Feminist theory 9, 25, 28, 144, 171
Folbre, Nancy 11, 36–37
Fraser, Nancy 37–38

Gaard, Greta 112
Gender 3, 4, 5–10, 18–19, 26–29, 32, 36, 38, 44, 50–53, 57–59, 79, 83, 90, 92, 95–96, 101, 109, 110, 112, 114, 120–124, 136, 137, 139, 148, 150–154, 158, 160, 165, 168–169, 171, 175, 179–180
Gibson-Graham, J.K. 28, 75, 119, 124–126, 130, 145–147, 178
Global North 18–20, 24, 28, 32, 36–39, 48, 85, 90, 95, 101, 145–146, 148, 153–154, 164, 167, 171
Global South 11, 18–20, 24, 28, 31, 36–38, 48, 57, 85–92, 148, 153–154, 168, 171
Globalisation 165, 167

Haraway, Donna 15, 16, 17, 24, 29, 91, 92–97, 105, 115, 118, 175
Harcourt, Wendy 36, 44, 90, 93, 150, 175, 177, 180
Hartmann, Betsy 16, 89, 92

Healing 70, 73–75, 110, 135, 138, 154, 155, 161
Heteronormativity 112, 141, 178
Hope 14, 28, 33, 35, 46, 52, 56, 61, 63, 67, 68, 73, 75, 95, 101, 108, 114, 117–118, 121, 123, 125, 135, 148, 151–152, 155, 159, 165, 170

Indigenous peoples 24, 27, 68–69, 70–73, 134, 161–163
Interspecies 13, 25, 27, 51, 96–99, 100, 102–118, 150, 160, 175

Justice 18, 25, 27, 33, 51–61, 65–69, 73, 87, 88–93, 95–97, 104–106, 108–111, 114, 117, 119, 120, 122, 129, 135–141, 152, 154–159, 168, 173–174, 176, 181

Kimmerer Wall, Robin 73–75, 130, 156–157, 174
Kinning 15–16, 80, 89, 94, 96
Krasny, Elke 11, 33, 35, 46, 49, 143, 172–173, 179

Lake 1–9, 15, 18, 74, 96, 132–133, 165
Love 9, 10, 16, 17, 24, 36, 64, 75, 81, 82, 96, 99, 103, 108, 110–111, 118, 124, 139, 141, 156, 159, 162, 165

Meal cultures 4–8
Mezzadri, Alexandra 31, 38
Migrants 42, 47, 54, 172
More-than-human 12–13, 15–16, 23–24, 28, 29, 61, 70, 75, 97–98, 100–103, 105–110, 112–113, 115–118, 123, 125, 130, 133, 145–146, 156, 159–161, 176
Murphy, Michelle 37, 144, 179
Mutuality 72, 133

Nature 1, 13, 15, 26, 28, 27, 44, 53, 54, 58–64, 66, 72, 74, 76, 91–92, 101, 103, 105, 114–115, 130, 137, 156, 158, 162, 174, 180

Natureculture 103
Neoliberal 13, 26, 50, 56, 88, 108, 141, 152, 157, 158, 169
Nurture 68, 70, 72, 117, 131, 139

Ojeda, Diana 38, 75, 92, 160

Patriarchy 57, 85, 147
Piepzna-Samarasinha, Leah 111, 140–141
Plants 14–18, 27, 54, 55, 61, 66, 70, 73, 96, 99–104, 108, 115, 132, 156, 165
Plumwood, Val 12, 14, 55, 61–66, 69, 115–117, 174
Population 16, 27, 37, 45, 79, 80, 84–93, 97, 110, 140, 174–175
Postdevelopment 21, 25, 28, 127–128
Power 3, 18–19, 24–28, 56, 67, 76, 88, 90, 92–93, 96, 97, 101, 113, 122, 130, 140, 144, 146, 148, 154, 160–162, 168, 171
Puig de la Bellacasa, Maria 18, 23–24, 100, 103–105, 108, 117, 134, 175

Queer 14, 28, 97, 101–102, 109–114, 116–119, 135, 140, 142, 151, 160, 165, 175, 176

Race 4, 9, 16–17, 23, 26, 36–38, 79, 83, 87–90, 94–98, 110, 118, 160, 165, 171, 175
Rai, Shireen 38
Reciprocity 24–27, 73, 75, 119, 130, 138, 158, 160–161
Relationality 20, 65, 76, 104, 161
Reproductive rights 19, 20, 89–90, 94, 174, 175
Resistance 57, 61, 132, 134, 138–141, 155, 162–165, 169, 173, 182

Sandilands, Catriona 14, 18, 100–105
Sasser, Jade 16, 87–88, 91–95

Sexuality 90, 101, 148, 150, 165, 169, 171, 175, 176
Shiva, Vandana 14, 57, 173, 182
Singh, Neera 21, 24, 130, 173–174
Social reproduction 24–26, 31, 32, 39, 51, 60, 77, 79, 93, 130, 136, 141, 169, 181
Soils 17, 58, 61, 71, 99, 100–106, 160, 174–176
Solidarity 32, 38, 46, 48, 56, 75, 92, 95, 114, 120–122, 125, 129–131, 135, 146, 158–160, 163, 165, 171, 181
Solnit, Rebecca 146, 165
Stories x, 1–7, 12–14, 20, 24, 25–26, 28, 32, 35, 39, 60–64, 69–74, 81, 83, 86, 97, 99, 106–107, 124, 138, 144–148, 150, 152, 158, 161–162, 165–166, 182

Teaching 9, 21–23, 62, 67, 73, 146–148, 149–153, 155–158, 161, 164, 168, 174–175, 180–181
Todd, Zoe 24
Toxicity 110, 113–114, 116, 118, 175
Trans movements 111–113, 141, 142, 162, 165, 179
Transformation 22, 39, 44, 46, 86, 124, 125, 130, 134, 136, 143–144, 152, 162–163
Tronto, Joan 11, 23, 31, 33, 36–37, 48, 53, 143, 159–161, 173
Tsing, Anna 18, 24, 99, 100–101, 105, 107, 108, 175

Vulnerability 28, 33, 134–135, 151–154, 156, 160

WEGO 12, 58, 131, 171–172, 174, 176, 179, 182

Zechner, Manuela 21, 46, 48–49, 134–135, 172–173, 177, 178, 181